SCARS & STAINS

Lessons from Intensive Care

Mark ZY Tan

BENNION
KEARNY

First published in 2024 by Bennion Kearny

Woodside, Oakamoor, ST10 3AE

www.BennionKearny.com

ISBN: 9781915855299

Acknowledgements

Intensive care is a work of frequent delicate balances, of sometimes thankless success, and occasional catastrophic mistakes. Unlike seasoned veterans, though, intensivists do not wear our scars proudly. For our scars are but an abrasion compared to the wounds experienced by our patients. Despite this, most ICU survivors are grateful for the care they have received and would make the same decision if they were to be in a similar situation. I, therefore, must acknowledge the suffering, the deaths, and the renewed lives of the many patients I have cared for. You have taught me more than any textbook can, and I consider my work a privilege.

I've had the honour of working alongside and learning from some of the most astute clinicians and doctors. Those who manage to strike a balance between the science and art of medicine are perhaps the finest. They challenge without offending, guide without forcing, encourage exploration without being reckless, model a humble and quiet confidence, cut with care, pierce with precision, comfort when called upon, and constantly perform with elegance and grace. They love their job, love their patients, and love their colleagues. Love and appreciation to Anna Szypula and the QE gang, Ed Cheong, Pete Young, Nicola Jones, Steve Benington, Francis Andrews, Neil Sutcliffe, Emily Shardlow, Sarah Clarke, Chris Booth, Geraint Briggs, and many other colleagues.

Thanks to Anna Szypula and the QE gang for being such inspirations, Aj Eusuf for encouraging and supporting me through training, Sarah Thornton for guidance, wisdom, and the cheeky way of nudging me toward academia. Thanks, Cliff Shelton, for being an academic mentor, and Paul Dark for believing in my somewhat unusual set of interests, channelling my efforts, and supervising me through the fellowship (which also gave me space to solidify some ideas in this book).

The voices, sounds, notes, and rhythms of my teachers and fellow artists ring out across this book. The decades of practising, rehearsing, and performing are hopefully not wasted – these words, the spaces between them, and the lingering feelings after each story, are a testament to your influence in my life. Thanks to Mario Serio, Derek Tan, Karen Yeo, Jordan Wei, Sing Lim, Sinclair Ang, Joanna Dong (and Jitterbug Swingapore), Brian Chirnside (and ACS(I) drama friends), Debbie Tan, David Lim, Karl Su, Debra Lam (and the RJC jazz band gang), Noel Tredinnick, Tim Baldwin, Daniel Woolley, the Cavaliers (and other ASO musicians), Ray Liu, Chaz Keiderling, Simon Wray (and the Boogie Inferno gang), and Amy Bowles.

Thank you, James at Bennion Kearny, for believing in me and my writing, for your bravery in publishing the ideas in this book, for your honesty, openness, and hard work. For critical feedback, thanks to Anna Sutherland, Anna Bishop, Heather HB, Kahfoon Gillespie, Aoife Abbey and ICM journal, Hektoen International, The Intima, and the Society of Medical Writers. Thanks also for permission to reuse some pieces.

Thank you Philip Billson and the Daily Service staff for supporting me and producing the services on BBC Radio 4. Dan Tierney for reaching out, believing in me, and producing *A Letter to Lydia* for the Lent Talks in 2021. I certainly did not, and still do not, fit into the brief of "six people well known in their fields". Thank you Andrew Goh and the Impact Southeast Asia staff for helping me nourish and maintain my roots.

A particular mention to Giskin Day and David Murphy. Medical humanities was perhaps the most insightful module at Imperial College London. When I was initially disappointed by the rejection of my application to enrol on the module, it was David who advocated and appealed for me. I still remember the words he wrote in the appeal: "[the module] could almost have been designed specifically for him." Giskin then welcomed me to her course, where I got a chance to visit the national gallery and diagnose pathologies in Renaissance art (that formed my first two publications), sculpt anatomy using clay, utilise my drama skills to "perform" medicine, and criticise single-use surgical instruments using a dramatic and unwieldy art installation. She then directed me to avenues for initial publications in medical humanities, discussed ideas about this book, and provided very positive feedback.

Ian and Michelle, thank you for supporting me and always being there (albeit usually late), for the deep philosophical debates and the frivolous gossip, for the shared interests and the opposing views, the drama, dance, theology, food, games, and everything in between. To many more years, my dear friends.

Shawn, you came after me but have, in many ways, gone before me. You read, wrote, published, and shared your experiences with me. I have learnt much from your critical eye, your broad knowledge, your feedback, and your friendship. Even though we don't see each other very often, I love you very much. Mummy, Daddy, your sacrifices have provided me with the wide range of experiences that have shaped my views, beliefs, and convictions. They have informed the book as much as my patients and colleagues have. Thank you for your unwavering support, critical eyes, encouraging words, and love in action. Mummy, when you wrote and published *Cancer and the Bronze Serpent*, it inspired me to explore publishing this book more seriously. To Annemarie, Miriam, and Lydia, you have given me hope during times when I had little. May this book bring you just a fraction of the hope you bring to me, and point you to the source of all Hope, whether in life, or in death.

Note on Confidentiality

As an anaesthetist and intensivist, I often write about situations which involve patients and families at their most vulnerable. Yet, a commitment to confidentiality is fundamental to medical practice. I have thought long and hard about how to balance the need to share knowledge and lessons with the duty to confidentiality. Although individual patients (and practitioners) must remain anonymous, and thus seemingly unappreciated, know that they have taught me more than I could ever teach them. So, I thank them for their trust, their humanity, and their resilience. The patients described in this book have been disguised to prevent identification. Any similarities that remain, therefore, are purely coincidental.

> *"Try to write as beautifully as possible, because well-wrought prose invites its own forgiveness"*
> *- Phillip Lopate*

Contents

Foreword

In my years as an ICU doctor, I've witnessed life at its most fragile and humanity at its most resilient. We often think of scars as the visible remnants of pain, but they are also proof of survival. And yet, for every scar that can be seen, there are countless more – those invisible marks left on the soul from experiences that shape us in ways we often don't fully understand.

Scars and Stains captures the delicate balance between these visible and invisible marks, reminding us that pain, healing, and growth are all parts of the same journey. Through the lens of personal stories, the book explores the depths of human experience, laying bare the struggles and triumphs that come from within.

I've learned that our ability to care for others is often informed by the scars and stains we carry ourselves. This book offers a reflection on that shared humanity. It's an invitation to confront our own wounds, to acknowledge the stains left behind, and, ultimately, to find meaning and strength in the process of healing.

I invite you to explore these stories with an open heart, knowing that they may at times be challenging, but that they also carry the hope of recovery and renewal. Much like the patients I have cared for, this book is a testament to the endurance of the human spirit.

Prof/Dr Matt Morgan
Consultant, Intensive Care Medicine, Cardiff University
Lead Clinical Editor for OnExam, British Medical Journal
Author of *Critical* (2020) and *One Medicine* (2023)

Preface

Dear Reader,

Up to 75% of all patients admitted to the Intensive Care Units in the United Kingdom survive. That works out to over 100,000 patients per year. Many of these patients would have died were it not for the advanced monitoring, interventions, and staff expertise in the ICU. During the COVID-19 pandemic, intensive care rose to the forefront of the media, but – at the same time – many ICUs closed their doors to visitors. The result was intense interest in intensive care amongst the public but a very poor understanding of what it looks like, or what it means for patients and their families. In that sense, even though the pandemic secured intensive care as a vital part of public health infrastructure, it also almost became a black box – a place whose inner workings seemed incomprehensible, unfathomable, and out of reach.

Intensive care medicine stands out as one of the most gruelling medical specialties, one of the last bastions of generalists' skills, and one of the longest training programmes available for doctors. Intensivists work with some of the most sophisticated machines, on some of the most unwell patients, and in some of the most emotionally volatile situations in healthcare. Where guidelines stop and suggest "seek expert help", intensivists start to operate. When one specialist disagrees with another, we are called upon to maintain balance. When families experience the shock and distress of critical illness, we can help navigate and provide support. With so much at stake, it is unsurprising that training in this speciality takes many years.

This book is the culmination of over a decade of training in the related specialties of anaesthesia and intensive care medicine. I have worked at the frontline of medicine, caring for the sickest patients, throughout the worst pandemic in recent history, in some of the largest hospitals in the country, and alongside some of the best clinicians. My journey has seen me cross continents, communities, and cultures – from the slums of Thailand to the wealthiest districts of London, and from the impenetrable jungles of Papua New Guinea to the labyrinth of large hospitals in the UK. Through these experiences, I offer a glimpse into the inner workings of intensive care, reflections on the human condition common to us all, and a view beyond life and health.

Anatomy, physiology, and pharmacology were my building blocks from medical school. They formed the basis of understanding the human body. Anatomy divides the body into layers, organs and systems. From the five layers of the skin to the layers of tissue penetrated to access the spinal canal for anaesthesia and pain relief, anatomy splits the body into manageable, observable components. Physiology taught me how these anatomical structures relate to each other to produce an intricately balanced and finely tuned organism. One that is capable of diving over 200 metres underwater in a single breath. Another that can thrive on the foothills of the Himalayan Mountain ranges some 3,000 metres above sea level – a place where most would suffer from mountain sickness. Physiology explains how humans perform superhuman feats and how humans can suffer from a host of chronic diseases from environmental, nutritional, and lifestyle choices. Add onto that pharmacology – the study of drugs and medicines. The ability to prescribe drugs gained from completing medical school was my set of trowels. With these tools and materials, I began to build.

When I entered anaesthetics and intensive care training, I learned even more about mastery of the human body. Applied physics gave me a detailed understanding of how the many machines on ICU work. The pumps, pipes, and porosity of a haemofiltration machine temporarily replace a failing kidney. The force, flow, and frequency of a ventilator can support lungs that are otherwise too fatigued to breathe adequately. Advanced pharmacology widened my arsenal of drugs to manipulate human physiology. I can make the heart beat faster or slower or make someone's blood pressure go up or down. I could stimulate muscles to move or paralyse a human completely. I can put someone to sleep, facilitate some of the most invasive surgeries, and wake them up without them even remembering when they closed their eyes. Point-of-care ultrasound gave me the ability to "look" into bodies, providing certainty that only the most astute of clinicians could muster. With these skills, I make diagnoses on the spot, instigate life-saving treatments, and block the nerves that transmit pain. I became an architect of health.

Built upon centuries of accumulated knowledge and understanding from the physicians of the past, and decades of robust, unrelenting research, intensive care has become perhaps the fortress of medicine, and a tall tower of healthcare. Yet, it is but ivory. This cathedral of science and medicine, although mostly filled with humans, often feels empty. Empty and devoid of soul and humanness. When it comes down to it, intensive care is far more than the machines, monitors, and medicine. At its heart is life support. Not just organ support, but LIFE. Life at its most fragile, most simple, most human.

In its simplest form, life support, according to the Resuscitation Council, consists of five steps of an algorithm: Airway, Breathing Circulation, Disability, and Exposure – ABCDE. These form an aide memoire and a structured framework for anyone to provide the most basic (and sometimes most effective) forms of life support. Yet, as Isaac Newton's third law states: "Every action has an... opposite reaction". Equally, the interventions in life support, whether basic as provided to someone collapsed on a street, or advanced as provided in ICU, have consequences. Some are easily predictable, while others are difficult to appreciate when time is of the essence and life is in the balance. In their simplest form, life and life support are also relational. They are made up of relationships between humans (and sometimes animals). They nurture, support, encourage, rebuke, chasten, criticise, and love us. Relationships give us life, provide meaning to life, and stay with us beyond the end of life.

According to bestselling author Sathnam Sanghera, written literature possesses the ability to appreciate seeming opposites when it comes to exploring complex topics. In *Empireland*, Sanghera manages to strike a graceful balance between the good and bad of British colonialism. Likewise, both mycologist Merlin Sheldrake, in his bestselling book *Entangled Life*, and botanist Diana Beresford-Kroeger, in her bestselling treatise *To Speak for the Trees*, take this approach in their respective natural fields. The former explores the many ways that research on fungi uncovers opposing theories in science, while the latter weaves complex scientific knowledge on medicinal plants with ancient Celtic wisdom of the natural world. Both emphasise how much we still need to learn and how interconnected we are to each other and the world. The same is true of medicine, and this is my way of marrying the known and unknown, the good and bad, the science and the art.

This book will explore some of the uncertainties of intensive care and life support while keeping the relational aspects of health and illness squarely at the centre of human life. It does not seek to explain all of intensive care medicine (for there is still much we do not understand) but does encourage people to care for others in simple, immeasurable, and intensive ways. It does not provide simple answers to life's questions, for such answers are almost never binary. But it can help to guide discussions around such questions based on experience and expertise at the most fragile times of life.

The stories may make you cry, and you may even be shocked at some points. There may be times when you feel overwhelmed by it all, as I have been many times throughout these experiences, and while writing them down. If this occurs, please do remember to put the book down and return to it another time. It has been crafted to do this, but I promise there is hope around the corner. I also hope the stories will help you think more deeply about health and illness, as well as life and death. And as much as I invite you into my world of intensive care through these pages, may you never need my help in such a setting.

Mark

1. Warm-up

Adapted from C.L Hanon: The Virtuoso Pianist

Airway

In the Resuscitation Council's courses, Airway is paramount. Whether for Basic Life Support, Immediate Life Support, or Advanced Life Support, checking and opening the airway is the first intervention candidates are taught to do after "checking for danger". The premise is anatomical. In an unresponsive, unconscious, or comatose individual, the jaw falls backwards, causing the tongue to obstruct the back of the throat. Air cannot get into the lungs, and without oxygen getting to the lungs, death ensues. As such, Airway comes before Breathing in the life support algorithms. Opening the airway may be as simple as lifting the chin or thrusting the jaw forward, but sometimes that doesn't work, or other measures are required.

The Airway section begins from the tongue and moves to the trachea in the neck, down to the smaller bronchi, bronchioles and – finally – the tiny pockets of alveoli in the lungs. The first chapter in this section contrasts three different methods of airway management in emergencies in three different patients facing three different situations. As scary as they might sound, these scenarios do not represent what happens during most anaesthetics. Today, anaesthetists frequently perform "advanced" airway management.

Every year, up to 20 million intubations are performed in the USA and up to 1 million in the UK.[1,2] Intubation is a very safe procedure for most people. Life-threatening complications only occur in 0.005% of all anaesthetics. During tracheal intubation, patients receive an anaesthetic agent, some strong painkillers, and usually a paralysing agent. As a result, patients don't recall the procedure. It is a skill that is well-taught right at the start of anaesthetics and intensive care medicine training. We practise it many times and have other tools at our disposal should the procedure become challenging. Throughout training, anaesthetists learn how to deal with difficult airways, too. Options may range from something as simple as a face mask (as in the final vignette of *A is for Airway*) to the more invasive airways like tracheostomies (in *The Perfect Storm*).

For patients who are known to have difficult airways, plans are often put in place before surgery or anaesthesia to ensure safe airway management. However, this should also be considered in patients with diseases likely to compromise the airway. In these cases, a pre-emptive plan to manage airway obstruction is useful for clinicians who might not know the patient. Such strategies are ideal, but between 80 and 93% of difficult airways are not predicted on initial assessment.[3] Fortunately, all anaesthetists are trained to manage such situations in a stepwise, methodical, and safe fashion.

Some people have a deep fear of waking up with a tube in their mouth. This may happen to patients who undergo a planned general anaesthetic and those who get ventilated on the

---

[1] Nadeem AUR, Gazmuri RJ, Waheed I, Nadeem R, Molnar J, Mahmood S, et al. Adherence to Evidence-Base Endotracheal Intubation Practice Patterns by Intensivists and Emergency Department Physicians. J Acute Med. 2017;7(2):47-53.

[2] Cook TM, Woodall N, Frerk C,. Major complications of airway management in the UK: results of the Fourth National Audit Project of the Royal College of Anaesthetists and the Difficult Airway Society. Part 1: Anaesthesia†. BJA: British Journal of Anaesthesia. 2011;106(5):617-31.

[3] Nørskov AK, Rosenstock CV, Wetterslev J, Astrup G, Afshari A, Lundstrøm LH. Diagnostic accuracy of anaesthesiologists' prediction of difficult airway management in daily clinical practice: a cohort study of 188 064 patients registered in the Danish Anaesthesia Database. Anaesthesia. 2015;70(3):272-81.

ICU. In ICU, the healthcare professionals are well-trained to provide clear explanations when a patient wakes up after a period on the ventilator. Painkillers can help reduce the distress during this period, and so can verbal reassurance. Usually, this process doesn't take too long, and once patients no longer require a ventilator and have the tube removed, they feel much better. Not every critically ill patient needs intubation, either. Many patients also receive other forms of breathing support, some of which will be explored in the Breathing section.

Breathing

The main purpose of breathing is gas exchange. The cells in the body need oxygen to function, which is obtained from the air. Carbon dioxide is produced from cellular processes, and gets transported by the blood to the lungs, where it gets expelled into the air at the same time that oxygen gets absorbed. Breathing thus requires the actual muscles and bones of the chest, the healthy tissues of the lungs, and the circulation of blood from the lungs through the heart to the rest of the body.

Intubation and subsequent ventilation form major aspects of intensive care. The stories in this section further explore some of the misunderstandings and uncertainties around being put on a ventilator. Like the Airway section, there are different degrees of "invasiveness" when it comes to respiratory support, from the mostly benign nasal prongs delivering additional oxygen to the nose, through the non-invasive ventilation used for patients with chronic lung disease, to invasive and mechanical ventilation. Different patients may need different support at different points in time, such as explored in the chapter entitled *85%*.

Fortunately, for many critically ill patients, mechanical ventilation is only required for up to a couple of days. In these cases, there are usually no long-term side effects. However, for some patients, ventilation may be needed for several days, weeks or, occasionally, months. For others, even mechanical ventilation cannot save their lives. Sometimes, this is due to the severity of the initial critical illness. At other times, existing co-morbidities mean that when one organ fails, other organs soon follow suit (see *The Three Sisters*). For the remaining that survive their initial few days in the intensive care unit, the ongoing need for mechanical ventilation makes them susceptible to a host of other complications. For example, most patients require sedation to tolerate mechanical ventilation. Longer periods of sedation usually mean muscles become weaker, patients take a longer time to recover, do not effectively clear their secretions, and suffer from reduced brain activity. A very small number of patients, after their critical illnesses, become dependent on a ventilator for the rest of their lives.

Therefore, the perception that mechanical ventilation is a life-saving intervention is not entirely accurate. It can be, for some people who require temporary support, but it is not universally beneficial. Increasingly, as the population, particularly in high-income countries, becomes more aged, co-morbid, and sometimes chronically ill, mechanical ventilation and respiratory support may become less effective and more unpleasant. In addition, there are complex interdependencies between the lungs and the heart, such that people with chronic heart conditions may progress to lung disease and vice versa.

Circulation

Ancient physicians, for centuries, believed in a heart-centred physiology. That is, the heart was the most important organ. The Greeks likened the heart to the sun of the cosmos, the ancient Chinese viewed it as the monarch of a city, and the Hindus imagined it as a foundation beam or cornerstone.[4] Yet, the assessment of the heart comes not first, not second, but third in the modern ABCDE (Airway, Breathing, Circulation, Disability, Exposure) approach to advanced life support.

In those days, it was sacrilegious even to consider manipulating the heart. But these days, we routinely perform cardiac surgery, which saves countless lives. This is not confined to high-income countries where lifestyle factors like smoking and a high-fat diet predispose middle-aged people to heart disease. In lower-middle-income countries, heart valve surgery can also help many young people cope with the complications of infections, allowing them more capacity for physical activity and thus

---

[4] Porter R. The greatest benefit to mankind: a medical history of humanity from antiquity to the present. London: HarperCollins; 1997.

opportunities to contribute to the economy and the growth of their communities. All these patients require at least a day or so of intensive care, where their vitals are closely monitored, their blood pressure is supported while recovering from the operation, and while they regain sufficient strength and cognition not to need the help of a nurse 24 hours a day. But while this peri-operative care (care that occurs before and after an operation) for open heart surgery forms an obvious part of intensive care, there are many other forms of circulation support.

For most critically ill patients, the heart can be accessed and manipulated through far less invasive methods. Drugs are often used to maintain a blood pressure capable of supporting blood flow to the vital organs. We use a whole host of such medications in anaesthesia and intensive care. Many of these require the insertion of invasive lines into large veins in the body to deliver the drugs close or directly to the heart. The skill of inserting these central lines is explored in the chapter *See one, Do one, Teach one*, along with some of the complications of similar procedures. Once in, strong medications help encourage the heart to pump harder, squeezing the arteries to increase blood pressure and even speeding up or slowing down the heart rate. Most of the patients in this book will have been given some of these drugs in ICU.

But just manipulating the heart is sometimes insufficient. The organs, muscles, and tissues of the body require blood. Blood contains the oxygen vital for the cells to function. It also delivers oxygen to the heart muscle itself and removes carbon dioxide. Catastrophic bleeding can, therefore, be one of the most traumatic scenarios in intensive care. Similarly, the most advanced heart support technologies may sometimes produce the most dramatic of miracles. This section explores some of these interdependencies through some incredible stories. There will be tragedies, miracles, and – at the heart of it – the human struggle with uncertainty.

Disability

The term disability – in popular culture – often refers to a physical impairment, or a sensory deficit resulting in difficulty for the affected person in doing certain activities or having equitable access in a society. In life support, it usually refers to the assessment and treatment of life-threatening neurological injuries. Three typical ways of rapidly assessing neurological function are pupillary response, the AVPU (alert, verbal, pain, unresponsive) scale, and the Glasgow Coma Scale (GCS). Pupillary response tests the reaction of the pupils of each eye to light individually and as a pair. AVPU is a rough score of whether you get a response to voice or pain or not at all. But in intensive care, we prefer to use the Glasgow Coma Scale, which scores three components (motor response, voice, and eyes). If more detail is required, full neurological examinations are performed, as in the chapter 万箭穿心.

Neuro-intensive care is often associated with trauma. Road traffic collisions, falls, and other accidents may cause head injuries, which in turn can affect brain function. These sometimes result in a range of sequelae, from no symptoms at all to minimally conscious states and even death. When the brain is concerned, outcomes are not just determined by the force of impact or mind over matter. Blood flow, oxygen delivery, metabolic state, toxins, co-existing disease, cerebrospinal fluid balance, and a whole host of other factors affect how one's brain may be affected by, or recover from, injury. For example, a stroke severely impairs brain function, even if not associated with trauma. Likewise, infections can also wreak havoc across the entire nervous system, affecting many organ systems (see *Flaccidity*).

This section will probably raise more ethical and moral questions than it answers. Two friends stand out as contrasting examples. Both Bernard and Johann sustained severe traumatic brain injuries in their youth. Both required craniectomies, which involve removing part of the skull to relieve pressure on the injured and swollen brain. Both spent weeks in the ICU and months in rehabilitation. Bernard never spoke again, was bed-bound for over 20 years, and was completely dependent on his ageing parents for his daily care and needs. Johann eventually recovered and became an artist. He continues to struggle with social interactions and speech but manages to live independently, earn enough money to get by, and contribute to society. Medicine cannot accurately predict the fate of Bernard or Johann on admission to ICU, nor can it reliably prognosticate all patients, as explored in *Chinese Fortune Sticks*.

Neither can statistics fully explain the individual circumstances patients and their families find themselves in after critical illness. The chapters in this section contain reflections on some of my struggles with prediction, prognostication, and persistence in intensive care.

Exposure

Clearly, life support cannot merely be summarised into five alphabets; otherwise, I wouldn't need over a decade of training to practise intensive care. Once immediately life-threatening injuries are addressed in the preceding four sections, clinicians can move on to exposure. This section encompasses checking for other injuries, maintaining an adequate core temperature while doing so, and the "Else". Anything else, that is.

Hypothermia, typically from submersion in water or exposure to the elements, is an obvious injury that falls into this category. It is serious enough to kill someone, but probably not as quickly as airway obstruction or cardiac arrest. Having said that, with sufficient hypothermia, a victim may eventually stop breathing or suffer a cardiac arrest. I have used this section not only to explore medical aspects in exposure, but also the more esoteric topics that weigh on the minds of intensivists today. Without giving too much away too early, I will say that the chapters in this section will take you beyond the ICU, beyond science, and beyond death.

Airway

2. A is for Airway

"Arrive, Blame, Criticise, Delegate, Exit."
- A satirical ABCDE

Another cardiac arrest.

Another surge of adrenaline, first for myself as I made my way to the ward, then almost invariably for the patient, too. After all, adrenaline is almost always used in the Advanced Life Support algorithm for resuscitations lasting more than five minutes. It causes the heart to pump faster and harder and is thus a useful drug for "cardiac arrests". A heart that is stopped due to a number of reasons may sometimes be restarted with adrenaline.

As for me, the naturally produced (or endogenous) adrenaline is a response to the high-pitched, ear-splitting bleeps of the on-call pager. It also causes increased blood flow to muscles for the short burst of exercise needed to get to the emergency, an accompanying increase in breathing, and more focused vision. All useful for dealing with urgent, life-threatening situations.

As both an anaesthetist and an intensivist, I would be expected to "manage the airway" in such situations. The cardinal "A" in the standardised ABCDE (Airway, Breathing, Circulation, Disability, Exposure) approach to life support. Unfortunately, such circumstances are highly stressful, frequently difficult, and invariably messy. Upon arrival, a rapid assessment of the situation must be done, followed by steps to secure and maximise ventilation and oxygenation. The team is often made up of strangers due to shift patterns, rotational training, and chronic staff shortages. As a result, I frequently do not recognise anyone on the cardiac arrest teams. This makes communication tricky. Equipment is usually lacking, and space is tight – all symptoms of an underfunded system.

Oftentimes, airway management requires me to stand at the head of the bed, which is usually pushed right up against the wall. I have to remove the headboard and push the bed out to get behind it whilst Cardiopulmonary Resuscitation (CPR) is ongoing.[5] Effective CPR itself causes movement throughout the body, which makes the process of securing the airway challenging (imagine trying to thread a needle on a bumpy train). In airway management, time is life. Without airway, there is no oxygenation. Without oxygen, life ceases. Everything ends.

Airway management in cardiac arrests frequently requires intubating the trachea or windpipe with a plastic tube from the mouth. A balloon is inflated to form a seal within the tracheal walls, theoretically protecting the lungs from foreign material and allowing artificial ventilation. It is as invasive as it sounds, and it is almost impossible for an awake patient to tolerate.

This cardiac arrest was on the surgical ward. The patient, a middle-aged woman who was also severely obese, appeared even more rotund because of the bowel obstruction she had been admitted with. For weeks, she felt bloated, then came to hospital after several episodes of vomiting. The surgeons had been waiting on her CT scan results when her cardiac arrest occurred, since her large habitus made it almost impossible for them to elicit reliable clinical signs of the paraumbilical hernia she had within her belly button. It contained parts of trapped bowel. Her dilated, obstructed bowel exerted pressure upwards – onto the lungs – which already struggled to keep up due to decades of smoking and obesity. Infection had then set in from the bowel segment, which had slowly lost its blood supply from compression. This rapidly spread throughout the whole body. Dehydrated from days, if not weeks, of covert obstruction, her kidneys suffered severe damage. All these culminated in her deterioration and cardiac arrest that Tuesday afternoon.

When I arrived, CPR had already commenced. The defibrillator was just being rolled into the room, but as I focused on the patient's face, it became clear that the bowel obstruction that led to her arrest would also complicate her airway

---

[5] It is a common misconception, particularly because of television, that CPR is highly effective. In fact, between 60-85% of patients who receive CPR in hospital still die. As author and palliative care doctor Sunita Puri writes, "The original studies for CPR having a 70% success rate were never replicated". As a result, there is often false expectations about CPR and what it can achieve for an increasingly complex, co-morbid, and frail population, compared to when it was first popularised.

management. At the head of the bed, a nurse and a healthcare assistant had put a bag and mask on the patient, diligently squeezing the bag and delivering two rescue breaths for every 30 compressions (as per the Life Support algorithm). Yet, inside the clear mask, greenish-brown vomit spewed out of her mouth. I quickly stepped in to take over, recognising that aspiration was inevitably happening. Each chest compression acted like a water pump, forcing vile, faeces-smelling vomit out through her mouth into the mask. Each forced breath was then sending the vomit back into her mouth and down her lungs. I had forgotten to put on gloves in the rush.

I grabbed the angled yankauer sucker and shoved it down her throat. There was none of the familiar, loud, slurping noises, but this was because of the sheer volume of liquid which filled the tubing. Soon, air was entrained into the sucker and the familiar slurps were heard. However, every time I tried to put the mask on to ventilate, more vomit spewed out from the mouth, straight into the mask and flowed onto my un-gloved hands. The defibrillator pads were now attached and CPR was recommenced.

"I need to intubate her," I said sharply, as I looked at the resuscitation officer. "Please get me a laryngoscope and a size seven tube." Those were the essentials; the rest could be acquired later. Ironically, or perhaps contrary to the laryngoscope's form resembling a scythe, this tool is a vital piece of life-saving equipment. With it, I could intubate the patient and secure her airway.

The resuscitation officer nodded, and as she rummaged around the emergency trolley, I prepared myself to intubate. Headboard removed, head positioned, suction still stuck into the mouth. Ongoing CPR limited the height of the bed, so I had to crouch. When the flow of vomit slowed down, I put the mask back on the face, hoping that the chest compressions would somehow entrain some oxygen into the lungs. Invariably though, more vomit started flowing, and I was forced to use the sucker again. By now, the white pillow on which her head rested had turned a disgusting shade of brown. Within the next two cycles of chest compressions and breaths, the equipment was ready, and I announced, "I'm going to intubate after the next set of compressions."

"23! 24!" shouted the foundation doctor doing chest compressions. The laryngoscope was already in my left hand, poised for action, while my right hand held her mouth open.

"25! 26! 27!" I started putting the blade of the laryngoscope into the mouth while her head continued to bob up and down with each compression.

"28! 29! 30!"

The compressions stopped, and the tip of my laryngoscope moved into position and lifted. The epiglottis came into view, then more vomit. My right hand reached for the suction tucked underneath the pillow. My eyes kept firmly on the target. More slurping noises. I could now see the two small arytenoid cartilages, which meant my target – the laryngeal opening in between the vocal cords – was only millimetres from view.

"Eight, nine, ten," came the voice of another resuscitation officer. This was a cue to restart chest compressions. But I was almost there.

"Give me two more seconds!" I shouted as I pulled up on the laryngoscope further, bringing into view the opening between the vocal cords. Gates that led to oxygenation, ventilation, and salvation. Gates through which slipped the plastic tube in a climax of airway management. Tube in, cuff up.

"Continue CPR!" I shouted, and the compressions recommenced.

I connected the breathing circuit and squeezed the bag. With each breath, a deep, coarse gurgle could be heard, along with a rumble felt on the bag. The patient had aspirated significant amounts of vomit into her lungs, and the fluid in her lungs now vibrated with each forced breath. I managed the airway, but it was not enough. I asked for a suction catheter and inserted it into the tracheal tube. Greenish bubbly fluid came back up. Her oxygen saturations were never recordable by the monitor. The irritant vomitus was now causing a widespread inflammatory response in the lungs, resulting in further fluid accumulation in the lungs, essentially drowning her in her own faeces and secretions, a horrible insult to the already fatal cardiac injury.

CPR continued to be ineffective, and after several additional cycles, the decision was made to stop.

Intubation was no panacea. As the doctors, nurses, healthcare assistants and porters slowly dispersed, I finally washed the faeces off my hands. I wished I could say "rest in peace", but for lack of a better term, it truly was a "shitty" way to die.

A is for Airway.

A is for Aspiration.

Aspiration: the process of stomach contents flowing into the lungs.

————◆◆◆————

When I arrived at the scene on the geriatric ward, CPR had already begun. It was 6 am – the time when the nurses were going around, diligently taking the observations of their patients – when 91-year-old Doris was found unresponsive. Accordingly, the nurse pulled the emergency buzzer and the cardiac arrest call was put out. He was a bank nurse who had never worked in the hospital before. He knew very little about Doris but told the first foundation doctor who arrived that there was no Do-Not-Attempt-CPR (DNACPR) order in place, so CPR began.

Soon, the rest of the arrest team descended upon Doris, who was initially given the label "asystole" in accordance with the flat trace on the defibrillator. None of her regular team were present, and so a treasure hunt for her notes commenced. As soon as I arrived, I walked to stand at the head end of the bed with a bag and mask on Doris' face and waited for the 30 chest compressions. I could not hide my scowl as I looked at her. She looked frail. Her skin, saggy and translucent, had lost its turgor through old age and dehydration. Her cheeks and eyes were sunken as her facial skin stretched and tented over the prominences of her jaw, cheeks, and temples. "Unfit for a haircut," came to mind, but my thoughts were interrupted by a loud, coarse crack on compression number 21. Her thin, osteoporotic ribs had just cracked under the stacked palms of the nurse doing chest compressions. I winced, but he kept his pace as he mouthed, "Ah ah ah ah, staying alive, staying alive."

"Ah yes," I thought, "the legacy of the Bee Gees ironically immortalised in life support courses."

"29, 30" he announced and then stopped.

"One, two," I replied as I squeezed the bag to deliver two breaths to Doris' lungs. But her toothless, gummy jaws made it difficult to achieve a good seal on the mask, and the resulting upward chest excursion was minimal. "Has anyone got the notes yet?" I asked as the chest compressions continued onto the next cycle of 30. I wished we could stop, but we were obliged to continue what we started.

By now, the vigorous compressions had displaced Doris' left arm such that it was hanging off the side of the bed, her flaccid wrist now flailing up and down with each compression. Her right was held down by a doctor performing an arterial stab to get blood for analysis. Over the next two-minute CPR cycle, I kept trying to ventilate Doris through the mask to avoid intubating her. This CPR effort was likely to be futile. Shoving a plastic tube down her throat felt like assault – as if dying wasn't sufficient – and we had to convince ourselves that she was indeed unsalvageable. Unfortunately, mask ventilation was ineffective. I had no choice but to use an airway device.

Instead of the usual tracheal tube, I compromised and used a supraglottic airway. This tube had a droplet-shaped cuff. Rather than passing through the vocal cords into the trachea, the cuff covers both the voice box and the oesophagus. With this device, I was able to ventilate Doris. Somehow, this felt to me less "invasive" than an endotracheal tube, as if the avoidance of penetration did not constitute sex. In reality, it might as well have been rape. Instead of a peaceful death, we broke her ribs, pierced her veins, and forced a tube down her throat. Doris had no chance of survival. The breath we forced into her did not give her new life.

I hated this part of my job.

By now, the medical registrar had found and read Doris' notes. He stood at the end of the bed and announced a list of her co-morbidities: "Frailty. Resident in a care home. Advanced dementia. Poor mobility. End-stage heart failure. Recurrent urinary tract infections."

All our suspicions were confirmed. We had indeed done Doris no favours. "Staying Alive" was no celebratory tune. The intravenous cannula was no lifeline. My ability to ventilate was no victory. Our interventions were all abominations. CPR was stopped. Doris' time of death was recorded as 06:32 hours, but we all knew it happened before the 6 am observations.

A is for Airway.

A is for Abomination.

Abomination: something which causes disgust or hatred.

———◆◆◆———

I did not feel like God as I walked swiftly down the long corridor to attend another cardiac arrest call in ward F9. Experience had taught me that our presumption of ability to reverse death in such situations was hubristic at best, or blasphemous at worst. Contrary to those medical dramas on television, most people don't simply "wake up" after a few chest compressions or shocks from the defibrillator. Yet, for the small proportion of them who do survive a cardiac arrest, our performance during those key minutes may indeed be a death-defying stunt. As a result, despite years of training and countless arrest experiences, I still feel butterflies in my stomach each time the bleep rings with that characteristic sequence. My anal sphincter subconsciously contracts, just like it would for a lie detector, betraying the calm persona I work hard to project. My jaw and lips often tighten as I make my way to each destination.

F9, Bay 3, Bed 7. The ward clerk pointed me in the direction, but this was unnecessary. I could clearly see the numerous nurses and porters standing in the corridor leading to the bay. Most of the team were already there. The cardiac arrest trolley – a red, usually under-equipped toolbox – had been wheeled beside the bed. On the right stood two nurses trying to insert a cannula. On the left, a doctor knelt, doing the same, their jobs made exceedingly difficult by the necessary chest compressions of CPR. In the middle, the patient was cyanosed (blue) and ashen (grey). I did not know his name, his age, or even why he was in hospital. It did not matter. He was now a label:

"Non-shockable rhythm."

"Commence CPR, 30 compressions to two breaths, rhythm check every two minutes. Adrenaline every two cycles."

Somehow, the label allowed the team to focus and follow a set pathway without the normal quibbles, delays, or disagreements characteristic of complex teamwork. Squeezing my way past the resuscitation trolley, I got to the head of the bed, where a hapless healthcare assistant had been allocated the role of Airway, a role she was clearly untrained to perform. In the adrenaline-fuelled frenzy, it seemed her primitive response screamed, "FORCE AIR INTO LUNGS!" So, she grabbed the mask, forced it against the face of the patient, and squeezed the bag hard. Unfortunately, this was, of course, entirely ineffective for ventilation. Instead, it collapsed the airway further, rendering all her efforts of ventilation moot. With each squeeze, oxygen billowed out between the patient's cheeks, as if blowing raspberries to mock her efforts. This was not insufflation; it was suffocation.

"Can I take over from you? Will you help me squeeze the bag, please?" I asked, to which I got a very vigorous "Yes!" This, I knew how to do. The label had been given, the algorithm would be followed, and the show would go on. I was no longer nervous.

Both my palms held onto the mask. My fingers grasped the edge of the jaw and pulled it up into the mask. The ancients called this "Esmarch's handgrippe", an appropriately Germanic-grunting, herculean-heaving, salvation-sounding manoeuvre to force the tongue upwards, preventing it from sagging and obstructing the trachea. At the next cycle, the two breaths were finally effective, with the chest rising and falling and the patient gradually looking marginally less like a corpse. After a further cycle, with sufficient oxygen and effective chest compressions, "non-shockable rhythm" began to show signs of life again – he took breaths, and a pulse was present.

It transpired that "non-shockable rhythm" had been given morphine for pain. However, his kidneys had taken damage from the urinary tract infection and dehydration he was originally admitted for. Morphine remained in his bloodstream and caused his breathing to slow down, which in turn reduced his blood oxygen levels. This then led to a cardiac arrest. With adequate ventilation and oxygenation, alongside effective CPR, he quickly regained consciousness. The simplest of airway manoeuvres made the most profound difference in this man's journey. Just as Esmarch's handgrippe saved many lives from airway obstruction during the early years of anaesthesia, so our interventions pulled him back from oblivion. My effective jaw thrust, along with adequate ventilation, was a kickstart to life. His breathing restarted and his heart began pumping. His spirit was restored in a simple breath of oxygen. I fought with Morpheus and I won. Perhaps I did feel a little godlike after all.

A is for Airway.

A is for Alpha.

Alpha: a name used to describe the Hebrew God.

3. The Perfect Storm

"The winds of change may rage tomorrow."
- Keith and Kristyn Getty

It went against everything I was taught in anaesthesia, but I did not know what else to do. And to be honest, I was glad I wasn't the one slicing open this woman's neck. But still, it was terribly uncomfortable. The only active dial on the anaesthetic machine was oxygen. No anaesthetic gases or sedatives. No pain relief. No paralysing agents. The years of being taught the "triad of anaesthesia" thrown out the window. The motto of *sedare divinum dolorem* (it is divine to relieve pain) of the Royal College of Anaesthetists had been conveniently forgotten. This was an exception, I was told – the perfect storm.

On the operating table, a gaunt, middle-aged woman. Hardly any movement despite the lack of paralysing drugs. She was breathing, but only just. The blue-grey discolouration of her lips and fingertips were manifestations of how little oxygen flowed around her body. Only several hours ago, I had been told about her at the evening handover,

"Just to be aware: Hazel Dobson on G5. She's 42. Head and neck cancer. ENT (Ear, Nose, Throat team) has scoped her. She's got almost no airway, and they are planning to list her for a tracheostomy or further surgery. If you get called, there's no way you'll be able to intubate her. She'll need front-of-neck access."

I've never needed to cut open a patient's neck to access their airway, I thought to myself. Statistics suggest that emergency front-of-neck access occurs once every 12,500 to 50,000 general anaesthesia cases. This means – statistically – that I should only expect to perform it once in my anaesthetic or intensive care career. Several films have dramatised this procedure by using household items. For example, in the medical drama *House MD*, Dr House performs a cricothyroidotomy on a patient suffering from anaphylaxis. In this scene, the suffocating patient receives a life-saving manoeuvre where Dr House jabs a hollow ballpoint pen sleeve into his neck. By doing so, air from the environment bypasses the obstructed upper airway and flows directly into the trachea and down the lungs. Very impressive. In the horror movie *Saw V*, a character did it on himself to avoid drowning. Several other movies have also featured cricothyroidotomies performed with various instruments. Heroic.

The reality is far more gruesome and unsatisfactory, according to a team of German researchers who put this to the test on cadavers. Not only are specific tools required (not just any pen), but an unacceptable degree of collateral damage was noticed, and the time taken to access the trachea would have resulted in permanent brain damage. Clearly, it's not quite as straightforward as the movies make it look![6]

Back at the hospital, we had finished the ward round by midnight, and there weren't any referrals from the rest of the hospital. Outside, the weather was atrocious, and my socks were still damp from the cycle to work several hours ago, despite my full waterproof gear. I sat down in the staff room, popped my meal into the microwave, started to brew a cup of tea, and put my feet up on the chair opposite, hoping my socks would dry slightly. The microwave pinged. I retrieved it, fished the teabag from my mug, and brought both food items to the table. And then my bleep went off,

"Brrrzzzzz. Beep beep, beep beep. Cardiac arrest, ward G5. Cardiac arrest, ward G5."

This was Hazel. Damnit. I put the lid back on my Tupperware box and left my tea on the table, then headed out of the ICU towards the four flights of stairs up to G5. The corridors were cold, and the rain on the roof created a drone. Sometimes, this drone was soothing and could easily lull me into a deep slumber. Other times, it was unnerving. I felt the latter on this occasion.

When I got to the ward, several staff members were gathered around the window of the ward's foyer. In the middle, on the floor, lay Hazel. She had climbed out of the window for a casual midnight smoke. The nurse, busy with almost 20 other patients,

---

[6] Braun's team did this study in 2017 where they got various medical and non-medical staff to perform cricothyroidotomies on fresh cadavers. With a knife and ballpoint pen, about four to five minutes were required to obtain successful ventilation. Only pens which had internal diameters of over 3 mm produced adequate ventilation. Most participants also took several attempts to perform the procedure successfully. Braun C, Kisser U, Huber A, Stelter K. Bystander cricothyroidotomy with household devices - A fresh cadaveric feasibility study. *Resuscitation*. 2017;110:37-41.

failed to notice her absence. But when Hazel tried to clamber back into the ward, she felt dizzy, fainted, and fell to the floor with a thump. This alerted the nurses, and they pulled the emergency buzzer.

Other members formed a semicircle around her. She was wet and blue, not unlike near-drowning patients. Soon, the rest of the cardiac arrest team arrived. The anaesthetist, Sam, got a breathing circuit and tried to provide some oxygen. I called the ICU and anaesthetic consultants – we needed their help. The medical registrar on-call summarised the notes. The surgical junior grade called his consultant. I checked back with Sam. Hazel was gasping. The obstruction to her upper airway meant little air got past. Sam said that he could only force a small amount of oxygen into the lungs. Her saturations were 87% on the monitor. We all knew where this was going – Hazel needed a tracheostomy. Any lower oxygen saturations and she would likely suffer a cardiac arrest – hopefully not before we got to the operating theatre. Various teams were mobilised. By this time, we had lifted Hazel off the ground and onto a hospital trolley. The porters had brought a couple more oxygen cylinders in preparation for transfer. Sam continued to clamp both hands onto the mask to form a tight seal on Hazel's face while a nurse squeezed the bag hard. With each squeeze, the chest rose ever so slightly – disproportionately little considering the amount of pressure applied on the bag. Drugs were given to see if we could reduce the swelling in the throat. Once we were ready to transfer, I called the operating theatre again. They were ready for us. We set off.

Anita, the anaesthetic consultant, met Sam and I in the operating theatre. The ENT surgeon and theatre team were also there. I felt way out of my depth. I didn't know how best to anaesthetise Hazel. Any drugs given would likely precipitate a cardiac arrest. Paralysing her would have likely caused complete airway obstruction. I asked Anita what drugs to draw up. She only mentioned the usual emergency drugs; we could draw the rest up later. Hazel needed a tracheostomy.

"Don't we need any induction agents? Maybe she won't crash with ketamine?" I asked.

"She's far too unstable. Just draw up some adrenaline and other emergency drugs," Anita replied.

"What about analgesia (pain relief)?"

"Her CO_2 (carbon dioxide) is so high she's essentially unconscious. It's perfect."

Perfect? A perfect storm, like the one outside, I thought to myself. I wasn't wholly convinced.

The lack of anaesthesia felt somewhat medieval. I had read the horror stories about surgery in the 1800s. In those days, before the discovery of anaesthesia, surgeons would be known by how quickly they could perform an amputation. Robert Lister was particularly well-known for his speed. He would get several medical students to hold the patient down with the leg to be amputated outstretched on the operating table. He would then get the patient to bite onto a handkerchief before he cut through flesh, sawed through bone, and inserted a few stitches, all within 30 seconds. His haste, however, came at the expense of accuracy at times since he once accidentally cut off not only a patient's leg but also his testicles. In another instance, Lister inadvertently cut off his assistant's fingers. After this, an audience member allegedly fainted and died of shock, while over the next few days, both his assistant and the patient died of sepsis, creating a shocking 300% mortality rate from a single surgical procedure. To give Lister some credit, though, he was also one of the first surgeons to make use of ether anaesthesia in his later career. Upon using it for the first time on a patient undergoing an amputation, the patient awoke several minutes after Lister's rapid amputation to ask, "When are you going to begin?"[7] I was not keen on repeating Lister's history.

Hazel's airway situation was as precarious as her lack of anaesthesia. But the calm portrayed by Anita and the ENT surgeon somewhat reassured me they knew what they were doing, even though – statistically – it was unlikely Anita had extensive experience with such cases. Sam continued to ventilate her through the facemask while the ENT surgeon prepared the neck. It was tilted back, or hyperextended, to make as much

---

[7] Thomas B., Saints and Sinners: Robert Lister. *Royal College of Surgeons' Bulletin*. 2012;94:64-5.

space on the neck as possible. The area was disinfected. We did a quick team brief. The scrub nurse had all the instruments ready and laid out. Hazel continued gasping. Her eyes remained partially open but did not fix or follow. We knew she had not responded to painful stimuli on the ward, so was probably indeed only semi-conscious at best. Her skin remained a dusky grey colour from severe hypoxia. I wondered if her brain would sustain damage from the lack of oxygen. Just as I had this thought, the surgeon put his scalpel to Hazel's neck. She did not flinch. *Semi-conscious.* More cutting. *Still no reaction.* Down to the trachea. I saw the cartilaginous rings. *Almost there.* A window was cut. *On the home straight.* A tracheostomy tube was inserted. The ventilator tubing was switched from the mask to the tracheostomy. Chest rise. End-tidal carbon dioxide. It was in the correct place. Paralysis given. Much easier to ventilate. Good air flow. Anaesthetic gas on. Asleep. Oxygen 100%. Dusky grey to healthy pink. Smooth sailing!

As the surgeon finished off the operation, Anita, Sam, and I discussed the implications of what we had witnessed. We knew that there was a significant chance that Hazel would recall some aspects of the night. One of us would find her the next day to explain the procedure and the reason for the lack of anaesthesia. We talked about the potential for irreversible brain damage due to the period of hypoxia on the ward. We also discussed more generally the ongoing plans for Hazel and the further surgeries she might need, along with some of the potential complications and issues surrounding that. Soon, we were ready for Hazel to go to ICU after the operation.

When we spoke to Hazel the next day after she had fully recovered from anaesthesia, she didn't remember anything from the night. She remembered looking at the awful weather out of the window and really craving a smoke. She remembered stepping onto the windowsill, pulling the hood over her head, and lighting a cigarette, but nothing after. No pain or discomfort. No recollection of the voices of surgeons or anaesthetists. We were all relieved.

In the past, tracheostomies were a common procedure in children, much more so than today. The pathogen then was called the *Strangling Angel of Children*, otherwise known today as

Diphtheria. The bacteria infect the upper airways, causing a film, or pseudomembrane, to form at the back of the throat. This pseudomembrane restricts the flow of air and makes it difficult for children to breathe. In addition, the lymph nodes around the throat swell up, making the airways smaller. Respiratory distress ensues before complete airway obstruction or suffocation. Tracheostomies bypassed the upper airway, allowing the children to breathe while their bodies fought against the bacteria. However, the mortality rate from tracheostomies then was also high, thus Diphtheria's nickname. Today, most children are vaccinated against it, although an outbreak amongst the Rohingya population in 2017 is a stark reminder of ongoing health inequalities across the world.

In ICU, we usually perform tracheotomies using a different technique called percutaneous tracheostomy. Instead of cutting the neck like the ENT surgeons did with Hazel, we use a needle to get into the trachea from the front of the neck. A wire is threaded into the needle, after which several dilators are used to expand the hole for a tracheostomy tube. This is performed under anaesthesia and paralysis, and requires at least two operators in addition to the nurse. While percutaneous tracheostomies sound less invasive than surgical tracheostomies, complication rates of both techniques are significant, at about 8-10%. Most intensivists will have been involved in or heard about severe complications of this procedure.

Hazel spent a few days in ICU before going for another operation to remove the cancer at the base of her tongue. She initially had a swift recovery, but owing to her long history of smoking and existing lung damage, it became very difficult to wean her off the ventilator. She required not only extra oxygen but also pressure support from the ventilator. With each breath, the ventilator sensed her effort and gave her an extra boost. However, when we tried to reduce the pressure support, Hazel struggled. She started to breathe rapidly and soon began to sweat. She became tired, and her oxygen saturations would dip. So, we had no choice but to increase the pressure support again. This went on for a fortnight, which was not unusual for some of our longer-stay patients. However, over the course of these two weeks, Hazel became more and more withdrawn. She engaged less with our physiotherapists. Her mood plummeted. She refused to get out of bed. We tried words of encouragement, threats of potential complications, challenges, and jokes. But none worked. Whichever way we tried, our voices were but onshore winds, inadvertently running her progress ashore.

As the team continued to urge Hazel to build up her strength, we slowly realised that there was another reason for her wilful paralysis. After weeks in ICU, she was numb not from the near-death experience when we initially met, nor from the cancer that was removed along with a large chunk of her tongue. She was not immobilised by fear nor narcotised from drugs. No. As I spoke encouraging words at Hazel each day and struggled to lip-read her many attempts to communicate with me, it became clear that what she had really lost was her voice. The cuff of the tracheostomy meant there was no airflow up across the vocal cords. Without airflow past the vocal cords, no sound is made. For weeks, Hazel was unable to communicate effectively, stuck in her silent world. Her sail was furled. Neither winds nor waves would move her forward.

So, we spent the next few days consulting our respiratory colleagues. Specialists in long-term ventilation from other hospitals were called, multidisciplinary meetings were convened, equipment was discussed, and weaning plans were put into place. First, we swapped Hazel's ventilator for one that could maintain a higher flow rate. Then, we set a schedule for deflating her tracheostomy cuff. This meant there would be airflow around the tube up towards the vocal cords. Finally, we put into place a new weaning plan that would prioritise "cuff down" time, and inserted a one-way valve that directs air up towards the vocal cords on exhalation. We explained all of this to Hazel,

"We start tomorrow. You might find your voice very soft and hoarse to start with. This is normal since your vocal cords have weakened over the last few weeks. But your voice should get stronger with time, and I think you will find it encouraging," the consultant for the day explained.

"I hope so," Hazel mouthed silently.

The next day, we began cuff-down weaning. We switched the ventilators around and deflated the balloon of her tracheostomy. We had an immediate reaction, but not talking. When the cuff was deflated, Hazel began to cough. While we expected this, Hazel did not quite realise the burst of sensation in her upper airway. Air began to brush past her vocal cords, and as she coughed, an actual coughing sound was produced, which was not there the day before. When she stopped, she turned towards me and tentatively asked, "Did it work?"

It was soft, raspy, like a whisper. Her ears piqued. She immediately stopped, mouth agape with the wave of realisation, and then started laughing!

"It worked! It worked! Thank you!"

The rest, as they say, is history. Hazel caught a fresh breeze of motivation with the return of her voice. With the wind on her cords, she once again raised her sail and worked with the clinical team. She continued to spend a further few weeks being weaned off the ventilator, and another few weeks preparing for the management of her tracheostomy at home. But equipped with her voice and under the guidance of our physiotherapists and nurses, she navigated every obstacle with ease, until she left the harbour of our institution and made it to the open seas.

"If the ship I sing doesn't also bring my one true love to me" - My ship. Music by Kurt Weill and lyrics by Ira Gershwin.

4. As Water to the Thirsty

"To be brave, by definition, one has first to be afraid."
- Robert Harris, Pompeii

Of the many gruesome deaths that I have witnessed, suffocation scares me the most. I might not be afraid of death, per se, but the process of being suffocated – unable to breathe – is frightening! The airways are conduits for air. They permit passage from the mouth and nose to the small, delicate alveoli of the lungs, which facilitate gas exchange. Without an open and patent conducting system, no oxygen would reach the lungs and no carbon dioxide would be removed. Rapid death would ensue, but not before a short period of sheer panic, what the ancients describe as *angor animi* (anguish of the soul). This pain, felt in the middle of the chest, is often described alongside the "feeling of dying".

In the historical novel *Pompeii* by Robert Harris, clean water was the spirit of the city. Pompeii depended on clean water for fish husbandry, agriculture, and hygiene. From the bustling markets to the sleazy brothels, water was at the centre of Pompeii's success. Underlying the availability of clean water were the multiple conduits and channels which transported water from the mountains into the city. It was the damage and obstruction of these channels which brought the entire city to its knees. So hidden was the engineering genius of the channels that the occupants of the city took for granted the clean water available to them at the city's main fountain. The book follows the young engineer Attilius and his band of unlikely heroes in their quest to investigate and repair the channels when the water supply to Pompeii started to show signs of failing. Little did they know, they would come across a problem far bigger than mere plumbing.

Patrick, a man in his 50s, came into A&E complaining of increased shortness of breath. I glanced through his medical records on the computer as I saw him being wheeled through to the resuscitation bay from the ambulance bay. But even without the notes, I could spot the tell-tale signs of Chronic Obstructive Pulmonary Disease (COPD). He huffed and he puffed, chest like a barrel from years of chronic smoking, which eventually caused irreversible damage to his lungs. He sat bolt upright, arms placed out on his knees like a tripod to maximise chest expansion. The classical tar staining was evident between his index and middle finger. The notes told me he had a tumour in his right main bronchus. This cancer sat close to where the trachea divided into the right and left main bronchi supplying each lung. He was waiting for an appointment to discuss treatment options, but his symptoms rapidly worsened over the preceding week, forcing him to come into hospital.

The nurses attached monitoring – saturations 90% on a maximum flow rate of oxygen. Despite receiving four times the concentration of oxygen in normal air, Patrick's blood oxygen levels remained worrying low. It was pointless trying to get a history from him. He struggled to speak even a single word. Each exhalation seemed hardly long enough to empty his lungs, let alone produce speech. Instead, on each forceful inhalation, he worked hard, with his arms propped up on the rails of the bed. His lips, blue-grey from the degree of hypoxia, pursed with each exhalation, while his neck muscles strained to pull the collar bones up, maximising chest expansion. The right side of his chest hardly moved, while the left vigorously expanded and fell with each forceful breath. The adrenaline surge from this acute episode caused his heart rate and blood pressure to rise. I placed my stethoscope on his chest. Left: coarse crackles. Right: Silence. Deafening silence. My mind screamed at the severity of the situation. In this silence laid his diagnosis, and through the silence approached an impending storm.

His right lung was obstructed. It was likely from the tumour growth but possibly from infective secretions accumulating into a mucus plug. I put both my hands on his chest, one over the front and the other under his armpit. With each breath, a thick vibration (or fremitus) rumbled under my palms. Then, during the exhale, I pressed hard and shook, trying to dislodge the plug. This frequently works in critically ill patients, particularly those who have pneumonia or thick chest secretions. There was no plug. Patrick got worse instead.

I will never forget the look of dread in Patrick's eyes. His pupils dilated further, and his eyes widened even more. The furrows in his forehead from the raised eyebrows gathered the beads of sweat from the exertion of breathing against an obstructed bronchus. His mouth was pursed to increase the pressure within his chest, keeping those airways open. His right hand gripped the rail of the bed tightly while the nails of his left hand imprinted my forearm as he clutched it for dear life, begging me to do something. I had taken my chance with a mucus plug, but this was the wrong diagnosis. Now, I could but stand and watch the saturations drop rapidly to dangerously low levels. He was suffocating to death in front of me.

Behind my professional demeanour, my heart pounded like his. With all the confidence of being an "airway expert", I never felt so powerless. Since the obstruction was deep in the chest, intubating and putting him on a ventilator would not improve the situation. I pleaded with him to slow and deepen his breathing. This seemed to help slightly, and his saturations improved. It was my window. I had to work quickly. A CT scan was booked to re-evaluate the tumour whilst I called the cardiothoracic surgeons at another hospital to arrange for a tracheal stent, essentially a semi-rigid mesh cylinder, to open the airway. We were concerned that without being able to lie flat, Patrick was too unstable for any surgical intervention. So cautiously and tentatively, I laid him flat on the bed. All the while, my eyes fixated on the monitor to watch his saturations. I knew that, at any time, his airway could fully obstruct, and he would asphyxiate. Reassuring him of my presence yet knowing full well I would be unable to save him in the event of airway obstruction seemed fraudulent. But somehow, he was able to lie flat, despite refusing to do so about half an hour ago when he first arrived at A&E. I took my chances and swiftly took him to the CT scanner.

The scan confirmed my diagnosis. The tumour had grown faster than expected, completely obstructing the right lung. The surgeons were initially hesitant to take Patrick to theatre and were equally concerned that anaesthesia would further compromise his airway and he might die on the operating table. I pleaded. Surgery was Patrick's only chance. He might die even with the intervention. But having now witnessed *angor animi* in his eyes, I did not want him to die in this fashion. The surgeons finally decided to take him to theatre. This was an extremely high-risk procedure: an effort highly dependent on impeccable teamwork. The anaesthetist would normally be looked upon to solve airway problems, but clearly this obstruction would not be corrected by normal tracheal tubes. Instead, the surgeon would need to use a rigid bronchoscope (a cylindrical tube with a camera on its end) to see the tumour, while the anaesthetist ventilates the patient through a tiny channel within the bronchoscope.

Patrick had part of the tumour resected to open the channel. After that, a stent was inserted to keep the channel open. It went remarkably well, and he was back on the ward the next day, awake and alert. His oxygen requirements decreased, and his breathing was dramatically easier. By all accounts, this was a success. However, despite the temporary relief that the surgery and stent brought to Patrick's breathing, we all knew that the surgery would only buy him an extra few weeks of life. He was likely going to die from repeated or related complications, such as re-invasion of the tumour into the airway or bleeding into his lungs. Indeed, over the next few weeks, Patrick grew weaker and weaker. He started coughing up blood, and his breathlessness increased over time. The tumour had slowly invaded the pulmonary artery supplying the right lung. The palliative care team had provided all the pain relief he required, along with sedative medications which controlled his anxiety, breathlessness and panic from the inevitable death which awaited him. Supplemental oxygen was provided for him at home, where he faded away in the company of his loved ones.

In Pompeii, channel obstruction caused chaos in the city. In humans, airway obstruction impedes the flow of oxygen and carbon dioxide, wreaking havoc on the rest of the body. In Pompeii, the repair of the water channel provided only temporary relief for the city's population. Despite regaining their water supply, the obstruction was a warning shot for a far greater disaster. For Patrick, temporarily fixing the obstruction allowed him relief from the panic caused by suffocation. Yet, in the end, he eventually succumbed to death through bleeding into his lungs. Like the inhabitants of Pompeii, the celebrations of the temporary restoration of the water supply were short-lived, up till the thunderous eruption of Mount Vesuvius in 79 CE. Thankfully, the various drug infusions and supplemental oxygen meant that Patrick died comfortably, unlike those inhabitants of Pompeii.

> *"I believed I was perishing with the world, and the world with me" - Pliny the Younger*

Breathing

5. Blues and Trouble

"…someday, someday darling
I won't be trouble no more"
- Trouble Blues by Sam Cooke

He was close to death when I arrived. Monitoring had already been connected, and the numbers on the screen confirmed the severity of his condition. But I didn't need the numbers. The rhythm of the beeping was rapid, double that of my own heartbeat. The bright lime-green "120" merely applied a number to his rushing heartbeat as it struggled to pump blood around his body. The corresponding sound from the monitor was at least a minor third below what I was used to during anaesthesia, and the baby blue number on the screen confirmed a dangerously low oxygen saturation level of 89%. A further high-pitched, handbell-like, high-priority alarm rang every second – dissonantly cutting across the flattened oxygen saturation beep – and formed an uncomfortable polyrhythm with his heartbeat. I reached out my hand to shake his.

Tar stains on his index and middle fingers. He must be a heavy smoker.

"My name is Mark. I'm one of the intensive care doctors. How are you?" I asked, already knowing the answer.

"My breathing… terrible," he replied, in seemingly broken English, between several breaths, by which time my ears had piqued as the oxygen saturations dropped a further two semitones. I had to work quickly.

"Oh, you don't sound good at all. Let me have a listen to your chest."

87% now. Clear respiratory distress: respiratory rate almost 40. Sitting bolt upright: maximising efficiency of breathing. Arms anchored to the rails of the trolley: increased work of breathing and use of accessory muscles. Gaunt facial and body features: is this cancer-related weight loss? Deep orange tan: manual-worker or cancer pigmentation? Chest expansion is abnormal: right side is hardly moving, left side is hyper-expanded. Percussion: left side hyper-resonant. Stethoscope: minimal breath sounds on the left. This is a pneumothorax!

41

"Novak, you've got a pneumothorax. A punctured lung. The lung has collapsed. We need to decompress it with a needle, then a larger tube, called a chest drain," I tried to explain, in a loud voice, using large hand gestures to mitigate the potential language barrier. He gave me a thumbs-up.

That'll do for consent, I guess.

I turned around and reached for one of the translucent drawers, picking out the biggest cannula I could find, along with an alcohol wipe. On the countertop were boxes of gloves. I took out a pair. There was no time for a local anaesthetic. I cleaned the top of Novak's left chest with the alcohol wipe, then unsheathed the needle, positioned it under the second rib, and pushed it in.

"Sharp scratch," I exclaimed as I inserted the cannula, knowingly underplaying the extent of pain he would experience.

Compressed air rushed through the relatively small calibre of the cannula, creating a deeply satisfying hiss of a life saved. But this was a temporary solution. The relatively small, hollow cannula would eventually act as a one-way valve itself, causing a re-accumulation of the pneumothorax. A larger chest drain was required to prevent this from happening, but this could take a bit more time. By now, Novak's breathing had improved, and he looked a little less grey. His oxygen saturations improved to an acceptable 94%, and he began to speak more than two words at a time. As I prepared equipment for the chest drain, I asked further about his history and the circumstances leading to his hospital attendance.

Novak was 47 years old. He used to be a musician, but in a Bojangles-like fashion, found himself smoking and drinking far more than he could afford and, once addicted, ended up jobless, penniless, and hopeless. He continued to play on the streets of inner-city London, earning only as much as would pay for his habits.

"What sort of music did you play?" I asked, as I pointed the eight-centimetre-long needle at his chest, with his arm held up and hand resting under his head.

"Blues," he mumbled, and then broke out in a deep rumbly coughing fit. If it wasn't the middle of a busy A&E, his pose could well have passed off as lounging and listening to music.

But instead of a soulful bend in a guitar solo, he grimaced when my needle twanged the sensitive nerves of the outer lining of his lung, the parietal pleura.

"Very nice. I meant blues, not the pain; sorry about that. I do blues dancing actually," I said, as I then inserted the guidewire into the needle, which would serve as a track for the actual chest drain later. Seizing the opportunity, I indulged what I thought was my own clever little explanation: "The lungs and their lining normally move together – always dancing. When the lung is punctured for whatever reason, it tends to shrink down, while the ribcage prefers to spring outwards. Less lung is involved in extracting oxygen from the air and people get short of breath. In a sense, our bodies much prefer a good blues dance than a silent disco."

Novak let out a polite snigger. I wasn't sure he appreciated my joke about silent discos, but the chest drain was now done. The circuit was connected to a rigid tube submerged in a bottle of water. On each exhale, bubbles appeared from the underwater end of the tube. When Novak's chest expanded on the next inhalation, the water meniscus rose several centimetres up the tube, but, unable to overcome gravity, the underwater seal effectively formed a one-way valve, allowing air out of the chest but not back in.

Another life saved. But there's something up with that cough.

My intuition was right. There was no sustained recovery, and only a couple of hours later, Novak's oxygen saturations started to fall again. His shortness of breath worsened. On the chest X-ray, the original pneumothorax had already started to resolve, but it also showed a nasty pneumonia on the right and further inflammatory changes to the lungs. They were filling up with fluid fast, and I was faced with no choice but to put him to sleep and onto a ventilator. I called a couple of colleagues to assist me and explained to Novak what was about to happen. Not long after, he was intubated and brought up to the intensive care unit. An ultrasound scan revealed the cause of his deterioration. Surrounding his right lung were multiple, loculated pockets of pus, also known as an empyema. The inflammation that resulted from the empyema had caused fluid to leak into his lung units. The antibiotics we had already started were unlikely to resolve such a collection, so, according to the age-old Hippocratic wisdom of *"ubi pus, ibi evacua"* (where there is pus, evacuate it), I got ready for another chest drain but this time with a far larger surgical drain, roughly the circumference of my thumb.

Novak's right arm was held in position up and out with his hand under his head. This exposed the area beneath his armpit, the so-called "safe triangle". With a scalpel, I made a cut in between his ribs. Then, a pair of tissue clips were used to dissect down past the three layers of muscles before getting to the pleura. An audible, dull pop was produced as the clip punctured the pleura, followed by a spurt of viscous, cream-coloured pus onto my gown. I was glad he was sedated. The pus oozed out and flowed down the side of his chest as I replaced the clip with my finger. Then, the surgical chest drain went in to replace my finger. By now, the stench of the pus had filled the room – a pungent and repulsive smell of dead cells and bacteria. Behind my surgical mask, even breathing through my mouth failed to mask the potency of the odour, until I connected the chest drain itself to the underwater seal unit and the system was contained. By the time I stitched the drain to his chest to keep it in position, almost a litre of pus had already flowed into the bottle.

With the help of the ventilator, high concentrations of oxygen, and the two chest drains, the monitor was beeping in far more agreeable tones and rhythms. Novak's oxygen saturation was 93% – acceptable, even though it required 80% of oxygen from the ventilator. His heart rate settled with better oxygenation and proper sedation. His blood pressure became less labile, and there was some degree of stability. My ears were appeased, but my mind was not completely satisfied. The speed of deterioration, the level of advanced support required, and the strange smell of the pus left me feeling like we were missing something. But according to the protocols, we had done everything we could for now. He was on broad-spectrum antibiotics, which would act against a wide variety of bacteria. He had had relevant initial X-rays and ultrasounds. We had taken further blood tests. Samples were sent off to the lab. The admission document was completed, and the relevant paperwork was filled in. We even asked for expert opinions from the respiratory physicians and cardio-thoracic surgeons. My job was done for that day, and I headed into the evening handover.

◆◆◆

After my shift, I headed into the city. I had missed the dance classes during the day, but it was the blues afterparty that I was looking forward to. As I approached the dance hall, slow, sultry blues music streamed outwards from underground. A crowd of people stood around the open ground-floor entrance. Some were smoking, many had drinks in their hands, but all were sweaty. I felt time slow down as I walked through the doors.

Inside, the musk of sweaty bodies hinted at the intensity of the dance, while the steady, swung rhythm seemed to slow my heartbeat, making my limbs and muscles feel heavy and fluid. Occasionally, high-pitched twangs of the guitar cut through the air like electricity. Accordingly, the dancers would break a move in response. Despite the individual movements of each couple, there was a unified sway within the entire hall, governed by the flow of the music.

I spotted Lucy across the room and waved. We had agreed to meet after my shift. I walked across and hugged her.

"How was the shift?" she asked.

"Alright, but I had to go home to shower after a really mucky chest drain. Stinky pus everywhere!"

"Urgh. Like many of my operations then?" she joked, referring to the peri-anal abscesses she drains in theatre as a general surgeon.

"Haha, very funny. Tell you more later. This is a good song. Wanna dance?" It was Sam Cooke's *Trouble Blues*.

Lucy and I met as foundation doctors. In those days, we stayed in doctors' accommodation attached to the hospital. I had a long-term partner in a different part of the country. But the shifts were long and instead of driving across the country to meet her at night, I stayed in the doctors' accommodation, where Lucy and I spent late evenings together chatting or practising dancing. That was years ago.

Lucy stayed in London for her further training. I moved away and married. Soon, the bliss of marriage was replaced with the grind of mortgage, childcare, and post-graduate exams. The

45

training was long and arduous, but when I ended up back in London for a short stint, I secretly enjoyed the temporary escape. Lucy and I promised to go out dancing together again.

Our secret shimmy. Covert chacha. Hush-hush hip-hop. Discreet disco.

She nodded and put her hand in mine. I put my right hand around her back. The fabric of her dress felt smooth on my hands. Her left arm draped around my neck as she put her cheek on my chest. Held in a close embrace, I closed my eyes and listened intently to the music. Cooke's soulful hum, coupled with the sparse and regular bass, made us sink further into each other's arms.

As the verse began and music swelled, I inhaled deeply. At first, I noticed the fragrance of her hair mingled with the scent of sweat. Then I felt her chest rise in unison with mine as we mirrored our shoulder rolls. I prolonged the inhale in accordance with a sustained note in the solo, almost to the point of discomfort, as our torsos pressed even tighter into each other. A downward glissando of the Fender Rhodes keyboard followed, and we both allowed our bodies to buckle dramatically. I exhaled quickly. She let out a long sigh.

Soon, our hips rocked together in tiny movements, an exquisite connection with each accent of the snare drum. The closeness and sensuality of each movement was enjoyed by both of us – the afterglow of the climatic keyboard solo. I glanced at the smile on her face through a mirror on the wall, and I'm sure she saw mine, too, as we turned throughout the song. I let her sit back into my right arm, her hips rolling in a circle with the peak of a phrase, before resuming the close hold. As the music slowly faded, our movements again got smaller and smaller. Each breath was matched. I felt her heartbeat on my chest, just as she felt mine on her cheek. A blissful moment of intimacy before a final dip. We then held each other in a long, tight hug.

We had several more intense and intimate dances before it was time for me to leave. I had another long day shift in under eight hours. Lucy and I arranged to meet at the next social dance. We hugged. She kissed my cheek, and I hers.

"You should come over to mine after the next social, for old times' sake," she whispered in my ear.

I smiled as I made my way out of the dance hall.

The tube back to my accommodation was almost empty, but the exceptionally noisy central line train muted my thoughts, or perhaps it was the alcohol. Lucy's scent lingered on my shirt, an intoxicating mix of perfume and sweat. I closed my eyes and inhaled. The music, the dancing, the embrace. It was exhilarating, a buzz I had not felt for years.

———◆◆◆———

Back at work about a week later, Novak was still in a dire state. His inflammatory markers showed little response to the strong antibiotics we had been giving him. He still required 90% oxygen on the ventilator and dangerously high driving pressures. His kidneys had packed in, so he needed the help of a haemofiltration machine. Strong drug infusions were required to maintain his blood pressure. The team was both puzzled and pessimistic. Then, a call from the microbiology lab came. Novak had Extensively Drug-Resistant Tuberculosis (XDR TB) in his blood. He had had this infection long before his presentation to hospital. What he put down to "smoker's cough" was, in fact, years of tuberculosis. But this was no normal TB infection; it was immune to most antibiotics. We had no effective treatment. This was a battle we had already lost, but not just several years ago when Novak contracted TB.

The microbiology lectures in medical school failed to accurately portray reality. Held in the Sir Alexander Fleming building, they clearly necessitated a cult-like celebration of his discovery of penicillin in 1928. Of course, we weren't told that resistance had already appeared within 20 years of discovery. We weren't told about irresponsible antibiotic use globally, from over-the-counter prescriptions for inappropriate indications (like my family insisted on for my frequent but minor viral illnesses in childhood) to widespread use in livestock as growth promoters, after which traces would remain in the meat products sold in supermarkets. No, instead, we were taught about all the different classes of modern antibiotics, with complicated names like "macrolides", "tetracyclines", and "glycopeptides". We were taught various drug targets, from inhibition of protein synthesis to bacterial cell wall disruption. This was medicine. We were the brightest minds. We could synthesise new drugs, manage chronic conditions, treat infections, and cure cancers! So we were told.

It turns out we have been dancing with death all along in a slash-and-grab, bump-and-grind, down-and-dirty orgy of collective irresponsibility. We had bred extreme drug-resistant TB with decades of antibiotic misuse, even though these drugs continue to be some of the most valuable tools in our medical arsenal. The adulterous affair of Novak's lungs with the invisible super-bacteria sealed his fate. All I could do was to make his death as dignified as possible, and so, as I put a blues playlist on his bedside speakers, and heard Cooke's *Trouble Blues* ring out, I prayed that, at the very least, our send-off to the heavenly realms would be as musical as he would want it. For Novak, the world and its pain, suffering, and injustice indeed "won't be trouble no more". But I knew it would only be several weeks till the next patient with another antibiotic-resistant infection came in.

I didn't go dancing with Lucy that night and instead took the long drive back to my wife.

[Winner of the Next Generation Short Story prize for the Health/Wellbeing theme in 2024.]

6. 85%

"The absorbance of a material is directly proportional to its thickness and the concentration of attenuating species." - Beer Lambert Law

I learnt very little about the inner workings of the pulse oximeter, otherwise known as the saturations probe, in medical school. While I knew that a normal person breathing air should have saturations above 94%, I did not know exactly how it was measured. Somehow, the little probe with a red light managed to estimate oxygen saturations through the finger. It was only in anaesthetics training, several years after graduating from medical school, that I was taught the importance of knowing the principles behind the pulse oximeter.

Working on the Beer-Lambert Law, above, the pulse oximeter emits infra-red light and visible red light. Much like how red and blue provide the illusion of depth for 3D glasses, red and infrared light get absorbed in varying degrees depending on the ratio of oxygenated haemoglobin and de-oxygenated haemoglobin, allowing a computer to compare these values and estimate the percentage of oxygen saturation in the blood just from a finger or earlobe.

The pulse oximeter only became widely available in the 1980s, after its invention in 1973 by Takuo Aoyagi. World War II had already accelerated the interest in oximetry as a way to detect hypoxia (or low oxygen levels) in military pilots. This was common at high altitudes due to the lack of pressurisation in the cabins, then. Hypoxic pilots would then lose consciousness and crash.

In order to measure oxygen saturation, the initial probes required calibration in the form of squeezing out blood from the ear or finger web. This accounted for the thickness of the tissue. Following this, blood was allowed into the finger or ear again, and the ratio of red and infrared light was read. However, this was clearly impractical when flying a plane several thousand metres above the ground.

Aoyagi, who died in 2020, initially aimed to use oximetry to measure the amount of blood pumped out of the heart over time: the cardiac output. However, artery pulsations produced unacceptable inaccuracies. Undeterred, he reimagined the "noise" created by arterial pulsations as a way to mitigate the need for calibration of the oximeter for oxygen saturations. By only considering the pulsatile part of the signal, differences in tissue thicknesses between patients could be negated. This allowed for the rapid, fairly accurate estimation of oxygen saturations in patients, just through an earlobe or finger probe.

By 1988, the Association of Anaesthetists in Great Britain and Ireland (AAGBI) recognised the importance of this non-invasive method of estimating saturation. In the first edition of their guidelines for minimum monitoring during anaesthesia, the pulse oximeter was featured as a strongly recommended component for continuously monitoring patients.

As many doctors know, there are limitations to the use of the pulse oximeter. As with many measurements in medicine, sometimes the exact number is not quite as important as the overall clinical impression. Thus, an oxygen saturation of 85% has different meanings for different patients and to different doctors. In a sense, just as was described for Aoyagi's manipulation of signal noise for this invention, the idiom of "one man's noise is another man's signal" stands true for this.

———————◆◆————————

Jack was in his sixties. He was a heavy smoker and lived with his wife, who was also a heavy smoker. Decades of direct and second-hand smoking had caused irreversible damage to his lungs, resulting in a condition called Chronic Obstructive Pulmonary Disease (COPD). The small air sacs in the lungs, dilated and damaged, become much less efficient at exchanging gases. Alongside that, his body had gotten used to a lower oxygen concentration in his blood.

I was called to see Jack in A&E, as the doctors were concerned by the degree of hypoxia they were seeing in him. He was short, stout, and obese, with rough facial features and folds of fat and excess skin around his neck. The prominent capillaries on his face revealed the chronic back pressure from the right side of his heart associated with high blood pressure through his pulmonary (lung) system. The blue tinge to his lips and nose was a worrying manifestation of the degree of hypoxia. He was sat upright, with his arms propped forward to enable the large pectoralis major muscles (and other accessory muscles) to assist in the expansion of the ribcage and thus the lungs to optimise ventilation. I looked up at the monitor to see his saturations at 85%, despite being on a fair amount of oxygen.

Mildly concerned with those saturations, yet slightly reassured by how well he was coping, I proceeded to assess him.

"Hello Jack, my name is Mark. I'm one of the intensive care doctors. How are you doing?" I opened.

"Not too bad!" came a chirpy, enthusiastic reply, which I did not expect. The ability to speak short sentences requires a surprisingly complex pattern and sequence of neuronal firing and muscular contractions. The brain, having received my question, integrated information to form an answer. This signal was then fired down via nerves to the voice box muscles. Coordination of these muscles, and those of the mouth and tongue, in phase with exhalation, then produce diction. Jack's coherent response thus gave me crucial information about several vital organs.

"How's your breathing?"

"Alright, not too bad."

"Really? You look like you're struggling a little. Has it been worse lately?"

"A little, but it's not too bad."

Astounding! I was not used to hearing such hearty responses with saturations in the low 90s, let alone 85%. Even in long-term smokers, saturations rarely fall below 88%. Yet this man was clearly compensating tremendously well.

The blood gas analysis taken by the A&E doctors also demonstrated a dangerously high carbon dioxide level in his blood of 10 kPa. This was double the normal level, and his already tired muscles had to work twice as hard to get rid of it. It was unsustainable. Jack would get tired. His muscles would produce even more carbon dioxide from the extra work they were doing. A vicious cycle would ensue, and he would slowly take smaller and less effective breaths. The carbon dioxide levels would then continue to rise. Eventually, this would obtund the brain, leading to further drowsiness and eventual loss of consciousness. Death would then ensue.

"Well, we're a little concerned about the low amount of oxygen and high carbon dioxide levels in your blood. Perhaps your breathing could do with a little help from our machines up in the intensive care unit," I said to John.

"Alright," Came the reply. It seemed as though everything was hunky-dory with Jack, but I wasn't sure if his brief answers were just a reflection of his personality, or a manifestation of his shortness of breath.

With saturations still at 85%, despite being on a mask delivering near maximal concentrations available in A&E, we rushed Jack up to ICU, where the nurses were much more familiar with the equipment we were planning to use: non-invasive ventilation (NIV).

The bed and several nurses were waiting for Jack as we arrived in ICU. One had already preliminarily set up the NIV machine. The machine was connected to a plastic mask using plastic tubing. The clear plastic mask, droplet-shaped, sat over Jack's nose and mouth, with a balloon seal around it to prevent air leaks. On the top of the mask protruded a forehead anchor. This was used in conjunction with two lower anchors near the angle of the jaw. Together, they allowed a cruciate strap going behind the head to be tightened, securing the mask onto his face. The visual effect is not dissimilar to that of the Batman villain, Bane.

The NIV machine provided pressure to help keep Jack's lungs open, while a flow sensor detected his breathing efforts and gave him further support for his breaths, allowing him to take breaths with much less effort. This reduces the work of breathing.

The NIV worked rapidly, as we expect for patients with COPD. Jack's respiratory rate slowed down, and he looked more comfortable. His saturations improved to 90% – satisfactory indeed for someone with severe COPD. Although he felt uncomfortable with the NIV mask on, he tolerated it well, seldom complaining about the snug fit. The nurses gave him regular breaks off the machine for sips of water and meals, but each time, his saturations would rapidly drop to around 85% again. Nevertheless, Jack thoroughly enjoyed each meal break as he polished off everything on his plate, from the soup starter to the cottage pie main and even the ice cream dessert.

At each ward round, the nurses never failed to comment on Jack's insatiable appetite. It humoured us that any patient would enjoy hospital food that much. At the same time, we were also giving him advice about losing weight to help with his breathing in the long term. It didn't matter that he was constantly breathless, or that wearing the NIV mask was uncomfortable; Jack seemed happiest eagerly consuming his meal. Besides, with his degree of COPD, there were few prospects for "long-term" health. Jack could hardly climb a single flight of stairs at home without getting short of breath.

Three days down the line, Jack's saturations continued to drop rapidly to 85% every time we removed the NIV mask or any form of oxygen. He was much more comfortable, having had antibiotics for the chest infection, which made his breathing worse in the first place, but his saturations were no better than when he came in. He was still talking in half-sentences, just as he was in A&E. We discharged him to the ward with minimal oxygen and saturations around 85%. He went home a few days after that, with saturations continuing to hover around 85%.

<hr />

Peter was also in his sixties, but his story was very different from Jack's. He was referred to ICU by the A&E doctors, who were concerned about his chest X-ray and how breathless he was.

"What are his saturations?" I asked over the phone.

"85%, on a non-rebreather mask. His respiratory rate is 40," came the reply.

"I'll be right down."

Like Jack, Peter looked surprisingly comfortable despite my initial rush to A&E. Indeed, he was in much better shape than Jack. His regular exercise regime showed in the toned muscles of his arms and chest, which were even more prominent when I saw him in A&E. I gathered that Peter was in his 60s and was fit. His weekly cycle mileage of 100 miles made my meagre daily cycle commute to work seem amateurish.

Like Jack, Peter was struggling for breath and using his accessory muscles in a tripod position. The pectoralis muscles tensed with each inhalation, as did the triceps as he anchored himself on the rails of the bed with his outstretched arms. Like Jack, his talking was only mildly affected, as he answered all my questions in short sentences. But unlike Jack, Peter had no typical signs of chronic lung disease. There were no tar stains on the fingers and no barrel-shaped chest. There was no wheeze on his chest or dilated veins associated with right heart failure. Beside his bed, his wife stood close by, clearly worried about how breathless he seemed to be.

I looked at the blood gas results. This blood test, taken from Peter's artery in his wrist, demonstrated that his blood lacked oxygen but was still able to clear the carbon dioxide produced by his body. His chest X-ray showed a nasty left-side pneumonia. Beside his bed, the monitor read out his observations. Heart rate 116. Blood pressure 102/54. Respiratory rate 38. Saturations 85%.

85%. The same saturations as Jack a week ago. In fact, the same saturations Jack had been discharged to the ward with. For a moment, I relaxed a little while taking Peter's history.

After gathering details about how he had been unwell and coughing for the last week, how he had no other medical conditions other than hypertension, and that he only took one regular medication, I got to his social history.

"Do you drink any alcohol?" I asked.

"Only a glass of wine at weekends," was the reply.

"What about smoking?"

But before he could answer, he stopped talking.

"Peter… Peter?!" I shouted as I shook his shoulders.

His eyes slowly closed, and he started to slump sideways. I shouted again, then I felt his pulse. There was none. Cardiac arrest! I pulled the emergency buzzer as I shouted for help.

"Sorry, I'm going to have to get you to step aside for the time being," I told his wife as I lowered the head of the bed to get Peter flat.

I knew the next steps very clearly: elbows straight, hands interlocked, palms in the middle of the chest, compressions at a depth of 5cm, 100 beats a minute. Within seconds, two other A&E doctors arrived, along with three nurses. In came the defibrillator, along with the airway trolley. That was my cue. I got two nurses to take over chest compressions while I went to Peter's head to manage his airway.

The ECG was an almost flat line, signifying that electric shocks were not going to be effective. Adrenaline was injected instead. I prepared for intubation as CPR continued. After two minutes, it was time to recheck the rhythm, and time for me to intubate Peter. The tube went past his vocal cords into his trachea. A balloon cuff was inflated, which secured the tube, and CPR was recommenced. 100% oxygen was delivered with each breath into the lungs. By the next rhythm check, he had regained a pulse.

I breathed a sigh of relief. He was clearly sicker than he appeared initially. Despite this setback, Peter stabilised very quickly once intubated. His oxygen saturations rose to 95%, and this was only with a moderate amount of additional oxygen. I spoke to his wife after this. Somehow, she was less shocked about the cardiac arrest than I was. I apologised for not recognising how ill he was. I explained that it was impossible to predict that he was going to suffer a cardiac arrest but that I was glad he was in hospital when it happened.

The cause of Peter's cardiac arrest was a lack of oxygen to the heart muscle. With half of his lung damaged from the pneumonia, he was unable to absorb sufficient oxygen. His heart had already been stressed for the last week since his symptoms began, but it finally gave up. The oxygen in the blood flowing to the heart muscle was insufficient for its demands. Fortunately, by controlling Peter's breathing, we reduced the workload of the muscles needed for breathing. By providing maximum oxygen, we were able to maximise the oxygen going to his heart muscle and so it restarted.

Early in 2020, around the time Takuo Aoyagi died, the "happy hypoxia" phenomenon in COVID-19 patients became a talking point amongst intensivists and respiratory physicians. They were observing many patients, usually young and previously fit, presenting in A&E with severely low oxygen saturations. Some were recorded with saturations in the low 80s, far lower than normal. Despite these low levels, these patients were noted to feel relatively little in terms of respiratory symptoms, such as shortness of breath, or signs like a severely raised respiratory rate. This was explained by several compensatory mechanisms in the blood and lungs, as well as the relative youth of the patients. Just as with Peter, they were able to compensate for the low oxygen levels for a period, until what was evidently a rapid deterioration, oftentimes requiring intensive care.

We stabilised Peter after this episode and took him to ICU. He recovered very well after his short cardiac arrest. On the ventilator, his oxygen levels improved dramatically; his pneumonia was treated with strong antibiotics. Over the next four days, Peter's oxygen requirements improved to the point that we were able to extubate him on day five.

I spoke to Peter the day after he was extubated. He remembered coming into A&E short of breath and talking to me. I told him about his brief cardiac arrest and the severe pneumonia that we had treated. He did not remember those adverse events. Aside from a mildly sore chest from the chest compressions of CPR, Peter recovered remarkably well. When he was discharged from ICU, his oxygen saturations were 95%, a dramatic improvement from the 85% in A&E.

As Peter left ICU, I remembered Jack, who was discharged just a couple of weeks earlier. Both had saturations of 85% in A&E, but with completely different clinical journeys. For Jack, I was tricked by what we normally consider a dangerously low oxygen saturation, when in fact, this was not far off his normal. 85% was the noise that I failed to filter. In Peter, 85% was a truly dangerous saturation level, a signal which, had I recognised it early enough, might have avoided his cardiac arrest, however brief. I clearly had much to learn about what Aoyagi demonstrated with the invention of the pulse oximeter over 40 years earlier:

"One man's noise is another man's signal" - *English idiom*

7. The Three Sisters

*"Death ends a life, but it does not end a
relationship...You live on – in the hearts of everyone
you touch and nurtured when you were here"*
- Morrie Schwartz

Once upon a time, there were three sisters. No thanks to their
genetics, their lot in life was tough. They were all born with a
hereditary progressive neurological condition. Sarah, the eldest,
was 59 years old. She was wheelchair-bound and dependent on
carers to hoist her from bed to chair and vice versa. She had had
two previous ICU stays for chest infections. These were due to
swallowing difficulties, which caused food to enter her lungs
rather than her oesophagus.

Having survived these episodes, Sarah seemed immortal
despite the weeks and months taken to recover from them.
Nevertheless, she could no longer eat safely, so was given a
gastrostomy tube to provide nutrition directly into her stomach.
Her recovery was never complete, but sufficient enough for her
doctors to provide non-invasive ventilation at night to support
her slowly weakening respiratory muscles. This machine sensed
her breaths and supported them by blowing additional
pressurised air into the lungs via the tight-fitting mask.

Sarah was admitted to ICU after a cardiac arrest. She had been
getting increasingly short of breath in the weeks preceding. In
fact, she was due an appointment to change the settings on the
non-invasive ventilation, but she never made it. Instead, her
carer found her unresponsive in her chair one day. She had
stopped breathing. The low oxygen and high carbon dioxide
levels, along with progressive respiratory muscle weakness, led to
a respiratory arrest and then a cardiac arrest. When the
paramedics arrived, they performed CPR, but her heart had
already stopped for a prolonged period before it was restarted.
By the time Sarah came to ICU, her brain had already shown
early signs of irreversible hypoxic brain injury. She would not
recover this time. Deeply unconscious, she was unable to breathe
for herself. We began the process of preparing for the
withdrawal of life support.

The middle sister, Sophie, was 56 years old. We learned about their common neurological disorder from hospital records. She, too, was wheelchair-bound and was dependent on non-invasive ventilation. I felt pity for her, but the longer we spent in conversation, the more I realised she didn't need it.

Sophie loved her life.

She was an ardent advocate for her patient charity, working to increase public understanding of the disease and provide a forum to support fellow patients. She held a stable job working from home and was well-known in her local community. She was a regular volunteer for local charities in town. Both sisters had risen above their diagnoses and freed themselves from the shackles of their sentences. This was the same determination described by Luria, one of the forefathers of neuroscience, when he wrote about progressive diseases, "the 'I' has vanquished the 'It'". Yet not unscathed, for the scar of near-death was worn at the front of their necks. Sarah had one, and when I noticed the same scar on Sophie, she proceeded to tell me about her own respiratory illness several years prior. This was followed by a several-month-long stay on ICU. It had taken her a long time to get off a ventilator due to severe muscle weakness. Against all odds, and contrary to the pessimism of the doctors, Sophie survived, but the episode did not make her stronger.

The youngest sister, Shannon, was the least severely affected. She was dressed in a plain blouse and jeans, walked normally, and required no breathing aids. If we didn't have her clinic letters and previous tests, we might not have known that she suffered from the same disease as Sarah and Sophie. Yet even Shannon was no stranger to healthcare. She had had several hospital admissions for chest infections and respiratory issues. As the most physically abled of the three, Shannon helped with her sisters' care and shuttled them to their appointments. Sophie and Shannon were accompanied by their cousin, Michael, whom they were very close to. No strangers to ICU visits, the family easily grasped the severity of Sarah's condition. They understood that death was almost certain and that the withdrawal of life support was appropriate and acceptable.

That evening, a call came from A&E. One that we hoped never to receive. Sophie, the middle sister, had taken a round trip out of ICU, halfway out of the hospital and then back into A&E. She had become increasingly short of breath and could not make it home. In A&E, exhausted, despite the non-invasive ventilator delivering extra oxygen, Sophie's oxygen saturations measured only 86% – a level insufficient to sustain life for long. Just by looking at her, it was difficult to tell she was working hard. Her muscles, weak and atrophied, were also replaced by fat. In combination, it hid the telltale signs of respiratory distress: an in-drawing of the rib muscles and pronounced straining of the neck muscles. Her chest, heavy with fatigue, barely lifted with each breath. But her face said it all. Dilated pupils. Profuse sweating. Pursed lips.

The assessment was brief. The discussion which followed was far more important.

"Sophie, it looks like you might be brewing a chest infection, but we are hesitant to put you to sleep to control your breathing. If we do this, I suspect you will not survive, and your muscles will become even weaker. You won't be able to breathe sufficiently," said the ICU consultant, Hugh.

"She's survived ICU before, ventilated and with a tracheostomy. She will survive again this time," protested Shannon and Michael. Sophie could only muster a nod and a feeble "yes".

"Yes, she might have done so previously, but she has deteriorated since then, and she has been dependent on the non-invasive ventilation and supplemental oxygen. If we put her to sleep, her body will take a further insult, and I fear she does not have the reserve for another prolonged episode on ICU."

"You don't know that for sure," they argued. Several exchanges of a clear difference in opinions followed this.

They were right, to a certain extent. It was impossible for us to be absolute with any form of prognostication. However, it was clear that Sophie had very little respiratory reserve. It was clear that she was struggling to breathe. It was clear that if ventilated and she survived, she would spend weeks – if not months – on the ventilator with a tracheostomy. Her recovery pathway would be prolonged. She would be prone to any number of setbacks along the way – any of which could kill her.

"We could try further non-invasive ventilation on our machines. These are stronger and can deliver more oxygen. Hopefully, this might help," Hugh compromised. I disagreed.

As we made our way back from A&E to ICU, we continued to discuss the ramifications of admitting Sophie to ICU for what I thought was a futile exercise. I argued there would be mission creep, and we would inevitably try to perform more invasive interventions with diminishing benefits. He agreed that was a possibility. I asserted that invasive ventilation would be a terminal event. He agreed. I said that we should probably discuss DNACPR (do not attempt cardiopulmonary resuscitation) when they came to the ICU. He agreed. I then asked why he was admitting her to the ICU when we had agreed on all these statements.

By this time, we were halfway across a long corridor.

He stopped, looked out the window at the hospital allotment, and said, "Oh look, they're planting the three sisters this year!" pointing to the sprouting corn, winding beans, and trailing squash on the ground. They looked strong and were already putting on fruit. I knew Hugh had a large garden, but I wasn't sure if this sudden change of topic was merely a way to make me shut up, a genuine distraction, or a coincidence with the clinical scenario.

Within a couple of hours, Sophie was brought into ICU, into the only bed space available, opposite her dying sister.

The day after Sophie was admitted to ICU, we withdrew life support for Sarah. Shannon and Michael sat around her bed, while I was sure her sister Sophie was also present in spirit from across the room. "In spirit", for Sophie was semi-comatose by then. Her oxygen saturations hovered between 85% and 89% despite 100% oxygen provided through the non-invasive ventilator. Her chest barely moved with each attempted breath, while the dangerously high pressures generated by the machine were simply insufficient to facilitate effective gas exchange. Not only were her respiratory muscles failing, but the infection had by now already damaged her lung tissue. Non-invasive ventilation was unsustainable, but invasive ventilation would no doubt secure and prolong her demise. The sisterly bonds, through intense grief, slowly suffocated Sophie as she saw her sister die. Shannon, distraught by the impending death of Sarah, turned all her hopes to Sophie.

I was then on a set of night shifts. As a junior trainee, I possessed much theoretical knowledge and a wide set of practical skills but had limited experience in complex decision-making. This afforded me the classic Dunning-Kruger effect of high confidence but lower overall competence.[8] Each night, I would ask at handover, "Does Sophie have a DNACPR?"

"No, the family are completely against it," was the invariable reply, accompanied by a brief debate about the best interests of the patient.

I sighed, "You know it'll be chaos if I have to intubate her overnight," pointing out the difficult intubation procedure and the skeletal staffing. Sophie was already hypoxic on maximal oxygen, leaving little time to prepare for a crash intubation – something I might be forced to do in the event of a cardiac arrest. It wasn't criticism in my voice but fear. Fear that, as the resident senior doctor at night, I would struggle to intubate Sophie. Fear that her severe hypoxia would cause irreversible brain damage (this was probably already happening slowly). Fear that she would die in my hands.

"Yes, none of us want to intubate her, but they are adamant that we should do everything. They have been distraught with Sarah dying just yesterday," came the reply.

"So, you want me to resuscitate her if she arrests? We all know that won't end well."

"If you have to, just do it for a couple of cycles."

---

[8] The Dunning-Kruger effect describes a cognitive bias where people with limited competence overestimate their abilities. It is often demonstrated by doctors who recently enter specialty training. While they have some knowledge and expertise, they usually lack a nuanced view of healthcare and a narrow understanding of the wider implications of their decisions. Frequently, one or more harrowing experiences produce some humility and a temporary drop in confidence. Further learning and experience then build both competence and confidence.

This was permission for a half-hearted resuscitation attempt in a Brazilian Portuguese *só para inglês ver* [9] type of fashion. I rolled my eyes. When this conversation repeated at the start of the next night shift, I got angrier. In my mind, it was clear that the best interest was to allow Sophie to die. To me, CPR would be considered an assault on an already half-dead patient. I was angry at the cowardice of my consultants. If the entire medical team agreed about a DNACPR, then why allow the family to "bully" us into not signing one?

Sophie was clearly deteriorating. She was barely breathing. The carbon dioxide in her blood, which normally accelerates the respiratory drive, had risen to the point of contradiction, narcotising rather than stimulating. [10] Her saturations hovered around the mid-80s despite maximal oxygen and high pressures on the non-invasive machine. Her blood pressure started to decline gradually. It was clear to all that she was suffering, and amongst the doctors that invasive ventilation would kill her. We were complicit in the prolongation of suffering.

Sophie's best interests were palliation. Yet, I felt the ripples of defensive medicine were slowly spreading, resonating and amplifying with each heated discussion to a tsunami, which would soon overcome the entire medical team with fear. The fear of one person's death was overshadowed by the fear of legal ramifications from the living others.

"This is bad medicine. It's not in her best interest," I protested.

"No, but neither is a lawsuit," came the blunt reply. My consultant was frustrated with my arguments.

---

[9] The British, who began the abolition of slavery around 1807, would not do business with countries where slaves were still traded. However, this persisted in Brazil, despite the inspections done by the British at the market ports. When these occurred, slaves were traded further inland to avoid being noticed by the inspectors. Thus, the phrase *só para inglês ver* (only for the English to see).

[10] Normally, a raised carbon dioxide level in the blood strongly stimulates the respiratory centres in the brain to increase ventilation, thus clearing the carbon dioxide. However, at very high levels, this normal reflex is suppressed, causing respiratory depression and decreased consciousness. This further exacerbates carbon dioxide retention.

I shook my head. I imagined the torture we would put Sophie through in the event of a cardiac arrest. Ribs would be broken during CPR. She would probably aspirate her stomach contents into her lungs. We might struggle to intubate her, causing more trauma and bleeding. We might have to cut open her neck if intubation was unsuccessful. Undignified, traumatic, unnecessary.

Somehow, though, Sophie survived the night. Two days later, the day team decided to intubate her. Thankful, as I was to escape the need to intubate her in the middle of the night, I could not help but wrestle with my own reservations about how the balance had tipped between defensive medicine and the patient's best interest.

Our feelings were right about the situation. Within a day, Sophie's heart rate started to fall. Her body was giving up. The more we forced artificial breath, the more her spirit faded. The machine was simply a poor substitute for the exquisitely complex human respiratory system.

Shannon and Michael spent hours each day beside her bed while we waited for them to accept Sophie's fate. After several days of what felt like ventilating a corpse, we finally all agreed that the ventilator should be turned off. By this time, I was sure Sophie's spirit had already gone to join Sarah's. Soon after the last breath was delivered, her heart slowed to a stop. After a short period of crying at the bedside, Shannon walked up to us at the nurses' station and said, "Thank you for giving Sophie a chance. We knew she was going to die, but we weren't ready for it so soon after Sarah. Thank you."

It seemed inappropriate to be thanked for switching a ventilator off after what initially felt to me like prolonging Sophie's death. Yet, her tone showed genuine gratitude, not so much for the medicine but for the compassion. Then I had an epiphany. My consultant Hugh was right all along. His answer was staring straight back at me daily as I walked past the allotment on the corridor. The three sisters were synergistic, a set of companion plants that thrived together more than they would if planted separately. Corn would shoot up first, followed by the beans, whose tendrils would cling to the corn stalks. On the ground, the large squash leaves utilised the sunlight falling through the tall stems of corn.

An exquisite harmony.

Consequently, when one sister suffers, the others don't do quite as well. Native American legend tells of three beautiful sisters who took shelter during a bitter winter. As a reward for the generosity shown to them by the community, they revealed their true identities as corn, bean, and squash. These plants, grown together, would produce far more food per area of land compared to monoculture and, in turn, feed the entire community throughout the harshest winters.

These relationships were the true centre of care between these sisters. The focus had long drifted from Sarah and Sophie to Shannon and Michael. In our minds, Sophie had already died several days prior. The relatives then became the patients, except it was not for physiological but psychological critical care. "Best interest" was, in this case, not bound to the individual but extended to the family unit. Had I not been so short-sighted, so focused on the individual, I would have seen the opportunity for care to extend beyond the confines of the bed and the walls of the ICU. Academic literature describes this as "post-intensive care syndrome: family". It consists of a constellation of symptoms and signs suffered by close relatives of ICU patients. These may include post-traumatic stress disorder, anxiety, depression, and other physical issues. In this way, critical illness affects not just the patient but the family, too, and sometimes for years after the episode.

Hugh had seen it – seen how this was a crucial moment which determined how ICU care would be remembered by the relatives. The clinical decision (or lack of it) was pivotal to how the end-of-life experience would live on in the wider family. Dying in intensive care has been shown to be many times more stressful an experience for a family than dying in any other place.[11] In his TED talk, Dr Peter Saul emphasises the importance of the conduct around death and dying, and poignantly says, "It matters how we die."

---

[11] Saul P. Let's talk about dying. TEDx Talks. Australia 2012.

We could not change the fact that two sisters were dying in the ICU just days apart. But we could alter our behaviour and approach to Shannon and Michael. If I had followed my narrow-minded decision to stop life-preserving treatment earlier, it may have resulted in a long-lasting loss of trust between them and healthcare. Besides, the decision to continue life support on Sophie was not purely altruistic. After all, I was sure we, as a team, were paying it forward. For, armed with the knowledge of the natural progression of the disease, we wondered when we might next see the last sister, Shannon.

"Of all the wise teachers who have come into my life,
none are more eloquent than these, who wordlessly in
leaf and vine embody the knowledge of relationship."
- Robin Wall Kimmerer on the three sisters, from
Braiding Sweetgrass

Circulation

8. See One, Do One, Teach One

"Docere", Latin root of "Doctor"; to teach

I started learning to play the double bass when I was 14 years old. I remember learning to keep my bow parallel to the ground and perpendicular to the strings while playing. This produced the widest, most open sound. Before my wrist muscles got used to the weight of the heavy German-style bow I used, my bow's tip tended to drift downwards towards the floor as I played. The result was a flimsy and scratchy tone. My teacher constantly reminded me to focus on either my right or left hand. She would demonstrate the difference in tone on her own bass, allowing me to realise how bad it sounded when the bow was in a poor position. It took weeks of practice to be competent at this basic skill. Either I would concentrate on depressing the correct area of the string with my left hand but allow my bow hand to relax, or I would focus on keeping my bow perpendicular but play the wrong notes. Such manual dexterity and coordination are a small part of what makes learning music so time-consuming.

How strange, then, is the hyperbolic adage in medical education, "see one, do one, teach one". It is not uncommon for us doctors to see a skill done once before doing it ourselves (under supervision). It would quite often then only take a few successful attempts for us to be left to our own devices or, worse still, teach another junior doctor how to do it. This adage applied not only to the basic skills of clinical examination but also throughout my training, even for painful, invasive, and potentially risky procedures.

As a third-year student, it was "see one, do one, teach one" for venous cannulation.

As a final year student, it was "see one, do one, teach one" for trying to puncture an artery in the wrist just by feeling the pulse.

As a foundation doctor, it was "see one, do one, teach one" for sticking a needle into someone's spinal canal during a lumbar puncture to obtain cerebrospinal fluid for analysis.

As a junior anaesthetic trainee, it was "see one, do one, teach one" for shoving a plastic tube down someone's throat, trying to avoid knocking out their teeth or cutting their lips in the process.

These days, inserting central lines is a routine, mundane task for me. However, it was only a few years ago when I was learning how to perform them. These large lines are inserted into central veins, such as the jugular and subclavian veins in the neck, or the femoral vein in the groin. They allow access for us to deliver potent drugs which would normally damage smaller veins. They are also used for taking blood and measuring venous pressure.

My first job in intensive care was in a small district general hospital that was unusually well-equipped, well-staffed with superb nurses, and well-taught by excellent clinicians. On my first day, a few patients were admitted to ICU. I got a chance to see the registrar, Jin, insert central lines into these patients as they were admitted. She was almost a consultant and had recently returned from spending a year in Australia working in a busy ICU there. The nurses liked her, and so did the rest of the consultants. She was a petite British-born Chinese, intensely sharp and incredibly smart. Back home in Singapore, we would have used the term "chilli padi" to describe her: small but extremely potent.

Before Jin inserted the first central line, she explained the relevant anatomy and potential complications to me. She then got scrubbed and laid out all her equipment as she described each piece and its use. Soon, she was ready, and the patient was positioned. I stood by her side, trying to remember the salient points as she raced through all the details. Before I knew it, she had inserted the central line successfully. I was amazed at how smoothly it went and how easy it looked, but I knew this was due to years of experience.

I had *seen one* inserted, and indeed, the next day, it was time for me to *do one*. The patient was a middle-aged gentleman who had just been intubated due to respiratory failure. He had developed sepsis from a severe chest infection a few days earlier and needed drugs to maintain his blood pressure. So, a central line was needed to infuse all the drugs effectively. Sedated and ventilated, there was no consent process. Unlike elective surgeries and anaesthetics, this was an emergency procedure in an unconscious patient. Jin was the registrar once again, but before she allowed me to do the procedure, I had to prove to her that I understood the anatomy, was aware of the potential complications, and could recall the steps of the procedure. I was thankful I took notes and re-read them the night before. She asked a barrage of questions, and after she was finally satisfied, we both scrubbed up.

After Jin and I positioned the head looking far to the left, we cleaned the neck with an antiseptic solution. This had an orange dye, which stained the skin the colour of a cheap fake tan. We then put a blue drape – with a window in the middle – onto the patient's neck before adding a sterile sleeve to cover the ultrasound probe we would use to locate the vein (Jin called it the "condom"). I then laid out the various pieces of kit neatly. Leftmost was the needle attached to a syringe. The next item was the guidewire, which would go into the needle. Following that was a thin, blue plastic tube tapered at one end. This was the dilator. A small scalpel lay beside it. Then, the central line itself, on the very right of the trolley.

I brought the trolley to my right as I stood at the top of the bed. I held the ultrasound probe onto the exposed neck and saw the target: the large, thin-walled, oval-shaped, compressible black blob, which was the internal jugular vein. Directly next to it, on the left, was the thick-walled, pulsating circle of the carotid artery. Deep to both was the apex of the right lung. I had to avoid these structures.

This was it.

My nerves had already been building, and I could hear each of my heavy breaths in my ears, making Jin's voice sound muffled. I felt each gush of blood through my carotids into my head, the same artery I did not want to hit on my patient's neck. My vision pulsated, and my throat became dry.

The ultrasound probe was in my left hand; the long needle was in my right. I was sure Jin could see the tip of the needle flail around with the trembling of my hand, yet she did not stop me. Onto and through the skin, I saw my needle as a white dot amongst grey muscle fibres on the ultrasound. As I advanced the needle tip, I simultaneously pulled back on the plunger, waiting for the gush of venous blood into the syringe. Meanwhile, while concentrating on the hand with the needle, my left hand holding the ultrasound had inadvertently put excess pressure on the neck, which caused the jugular vein to collapse on the screen. Like the incoordination while learning to play the double bass, my left and right hand struggled with the amount of force and subtle positioning while learning this new skill.

Jin stopped me.

I corrected my left hand, anchoring my wrist on the patient's cheek, but by this time I could not see the bright dot of the needle on the screen. I had to stop everything and start again. With my left hand anchored and my right hand at a correct angle, I pushed, millimetre by millimetre, until I could see the needle's indentation on the oval blob of the jugular vein. With the next millimetre, I felt the tissue give, saw the gush of blood into the syringe, and the bright white dot of the needle in the middle of the black vein on the ultrasound screen. I was in!

Syringe disconnected and wire inserted with no resistance. Next step done. We checked it with the ultrasound again. Correct position. Small incision in the skin, followed by the twisting motion of the plastic dilator over the guide wire. Dilator out, central line in. Then came the stitching. I was glad I had some previous surgical experience and was able to hand-tie my knots. That was it, my very first central line!

Behind my surgical mask, I smiled, glad that it had gone well. There was a deep sense of achievement, like producing a beautiful sound from a musical instrument. This surely was a glimpse of the deep pride surgeons feel from a successful operation, fulfilling their age-old maxim to possess the *eyes of an eagle, heart of a lion, and hands of a lady*? After all, spotting the white dot of the needle tip on an ultrasound screen filled with grey and black dots and lines could be likened to identifying a tissue plane with which to carry out safe dissection: the eyes of an eagle. Maintaining one's composure in the face of critically ill patients and performing potentially dangerous procedures in those so close to death must surely be lionhearted but gentle-handed?

Of course, I had conveniently ignored the small pool of blood which had collected on the absorbent pad placed on the pillow (evidence of the multiple skin punctures and my slow, unpolished insertion technique). But the nurse was not going to let me get away with my feeling of accomplishment. She was quick to point out the bloodbath I had caused on the absorbent sheet she had laid down in anticipation and made me clean the patient's neck before I left the room. Ok, maybe I wasn't quite gentle-handed yet.

<hr />

A few central lines later, I was gaining confidence and refined my technique rapidly, so was left to my own devices to insert one into a patient, Brett, with severe pancreatitis.

Brett was in his forties, rather obese and drank far too much alcohol for his own good. Either due to alcohol or gallstones, he developed severe pancreatitis. The systemic inflammatory response had made all his capillaries leak fluid, accumulating in various parts of his body, including his lungs. He came up to ICU for high-flow nasal oxygen therapy but was still struggling for breath, both from the increased fluid in his lungs and the pain from the pancreatitis.

After talking to him about the procedure, I scrubbed up and prepared the equipment. His head was positioned, and the whole bed was tilted head-down to increase the calibre of the jugular veins, and avoid air entrainment during deep breaths. This made Brett feel even more short of breath, so I worked quickly.

With the ultrasound, I saw the thin-walled jugular vein expanding and collapsing with each breath. I pushed the needle through the skin and, seeing the tissue above the vein tent downwards, the trajectory seemed correct, and I advanced. A tiny squirt of blood entered the syringe but stopped almost immediately, so I checked the screen and then, convinced I was still in the correct trajectory, advanced further. There was still no bright white dot of the needle within the vein. After what felt like a few millimetres, I looked back at the needle, noticing it was a little deeper than I had thought, so I pulled back, almost to the tip, to try again. Brett's head had been covered by the plastic sheet for a few minutes now. He became more breathless. I needed to get this line in, so I asked him to hold his breath. This distended the vein while I advanced the needle again. This time, blood came rushing back into the syringe, and I quickly threaded the wire before I lost my position. Finally, after confirming the position, I asked the nurse to raise his head again and lifted the plastic sheet momentarily to relieve his breathlessness. I was relieved, but this was short-lived.

About 15 minutes after I had finished inserting the line, Brett continued to feel very breathless. His saturations had slowly drifted downwards. They were 92% when the nurse came to look for me again. She had to increase the amount of oxygen delivered by the nasal high-flow machine. I had gone to request the chest X-ray to confirm the position of the line. So, with an uncomfortable feeling in my gut, I went to see him.

I was concerned that during my insertion, my needle had gone a few millimetres too deep, into the lung. I was right to be concerned. When I went to see him, the radiographers had arrived with their portable X-ray. I needed the chest X-ray not only to check the depth and position of the central line but also to make sure no other complications had occurred during the procedure.

After it was done, I looked at the small screen on the portable X-ray machine outside Brett's room. There it was. Instead of the fine, hazy grey lung markings on the right, a homogeneous black appearance lay under the top few ribs. There was no lung there. This was a pneumothorax. My needle had indeed gone too deep, puncturing the lung. This caused the lung to contract downwards and allowed air to escape into the space between it and the inner chest wall. The result was ineffective ventilation and gas exchange (see the chapter *Blues and Trouble*).

I quickly found my senior registrar, Chris, and told him about it. Chris was nearing the end of his training and seemed to always have a sensible solution to any problem. As he brought up the X-ray on the computer while I was explaining the situation, I felt mortified. Suddenly, a single word projected in my mind – INCOMPETENT.

It would not go away.

I imagined the word printed in capitals on my forehead. I had been commended on my technique several times while I was learning, but now, the confidence that I had gained from several successful insertions seemed to rapidly fizzle away, leaving me feeling naked and vulnerable. I felt sure Hippocrates was turning in his grave as I contravened the oath to "do no harm".

Suddenly, memories resurfaced from my childhood. Long before I learnt to play the double bass, I learnt to play the violin. I was about six years old at that time. I remember very clearly crying during many lessons. My violin teacher would criticise and shout at me for failing to practise. He would hit my fingers when they weren't curled perfectly on the fingerboard. He would frequently scold me for a suboptimal bow-hold. I grew to hate those lessons, and after a measly few graded examinations, I stopped playing the violin altogether.

Then, the fear of something else hit me. I had to admit to Brett that I had made a grave mistake. How was I to look him in the eye and tell him that I had punctured his lung? He had trusted me to insert the central line safely, but I caused a complication instead. Yet, Chris did not shout at me. He had seen it all before. He knew that this was a recognised complication of central line insertions.

"Don't worry, it happens to the best of us, Mark. Do enough procedures, and complications will occur. I'll sort it out," he said without even skipping a beat.

He was right. I knew it was a recognised complication, but it didn't make me feel any better. I still felt a deep sense of shame. I knew what needed to happen next. Brett now needed a chest drain. It would allow the pneumothorax to reduce in size and hopefully heal. But this was yet another step back for his already damaged lungs. It was another insult he did not need, especially since his body was already ravaged by pancreatitis.

Chris sorted out my mess. He spoke to Brett and explained what needed to happen. He then proceeded to insert the chest drain. Soon, Brett's oxygen requirements decreased, and his breathlessness improved. I just stood at the doctor's station and watched. My heart sank as I wallowed in my own self-depreciation. Mine was no heart of a lion. A mouse was more fitting, flitting between hiding places, afraid of others discovering that my competence clearly did not match my confidence.

For days, I doubted my skills, even in basic procedures. I felt my heart skip each time a chest X-ray appeared onscreen after a central line insertion. I read numerous journal articles about other complications, only to make myself even more anxious. Weeks later, I realised my place in the well-described Dunning-

Kruger effect.[12] I had fallen from my initial false confidence and my lucky streak of success.

I will never forget this episode with Brett, nor the courage which I had to muster the next time I had to insert another central line. Though my mind flashed back to images of the pneumothorax, and my heart raced thinking about all the potentially life-threatening complications, I had to continue learning and progressing through training. I had to pluck up the courage to carry on, yet not merely through my own sheer determination. Unlike my violin teacher, whose punishments prevented me from progressing, Chris's handling of the situation encouraged me to keep trying. His gentleness spurred me on, preventing the downward spiral into self-doubt. This was indeed a "minor fall [and] major lift"; profound lyricism from Leonard Cohen's wildly popular tune *Hallelujah*, using musical allegory for King David's subsequent rise to glory after his fall into the double sin of disposing of a subordinate through trickery and bedding his wife. So, through grace, I slowly regained confidence and courage.

———◆◆◆———

My journey to *teach one* was not quite as swift as some other procedures. It took a few years of inserting central lines and regaining my confidence to be comfortable teaching someone else to do it.

Hannah was also an intensive care registrar, just like me. But she had just entered the training programme, and coming from an emergency medicine background, what she lacked in invasive procedural experience – compared to her anaesthetic counterparts – she more than made up for in clinical acumen and diagnostic abilities. She asked me to supervise her putting in a central line.

As Jin did for me, I scrubbed up with Hannah and stood beside her as she prepared all her equipment. The patient, Irene, had been admitted for severe sepsis from pneumonia. Hannah and I saw her together in A&E and realised she needed intubation. After we had done so, we took her up to ICU. By

---

12 See *The Three Sisters* chapter.

this time, she was needing quite large doses of medications to artificially maintain her blood pressure. She needed a central line.

As always, the area was cleaned and prepared, and so was the ultrasound probe. We could see the target vessel on the screen, the internal jugular vein. Alongside was the carotid artery. This was the artery we were trying to avoid. Hannah began. Tentatively, she placed the needle on the skin's surface and very cautiously pushed. The skin of the neck tented downwards under the pressure, and the jugular vein underneath collapsed slightly correspondingly. A mild rebound of tissues restored the familiar image after the needle pierced the skin. Millimetre by millimetre, Hannah advanced the needle. I tried to keep an eye on both the needle in Hannah's hand and the image on the ultrasound screen.

"Good. You're getting close. See the indent on the jugular vein. But reduce the pressure on the ultrasound probe; it's collapsing the vein," I said.

Like me years ago, she struggled with the coordination of both hands needed to maintain a good image while advancing the needle.

Hannah aspirated on the syringe as she slowly advanced the needle, but there was no blood. The vein appeared squished on the screen, and I began to get a little nervous. I turned my gaze to the needle. It was in too deep.

"Take a look at your needle. I think it's a little deep now. Come out and try again." I advised her, fighting the urge to take over. Doing so would dampen her confidence. I was sure a knock in confidence at this early stage would set her further back on the learning curve. After all, it did for me with the violin. I stopped playing it for almost ten years (and switched to several other instruments before settling on the double bass) because my teacher severely punished me for minor mistakes.

Hannah's technique was sound, and her approach was safe. Besides, if the needle had accidentally hit another structure, it would have already done so. In addition, Irene's parameters seemed unchanged at that point in time. There was no rush.

I remembered Jin's coaching for my first central line and convinced myself to let Hannah try again. She retracted the needle and started again from the skin. I could tell she was nervous, but she did not fluster. As for any new skill, we both knew the initial learning phase would be tricky, and the central line is a core skill to master for an intensivist. So, I encouraged Hannah to try again. I reassured and supported her. She flushed the needle with some saline and started again.

Skin. Subcutaneous tissue. Vein. Flashback. She was in. The guide wire went in. A small cut was made. The needle was replaced by the dilator, then the dilator with the central line. Success.

By the time the radiographers arrived with the portable X-ray machine to check the position of the line, the nurse had already called us back into the room. Irene's oxygen saturations had slowly fallen despite an increase in oxygen delivered by the ventilator. Her blood pressure had also started dropping. I knew immediately what had happened, and a strange *déjà vu* feeling washed over me as I recalled my encounter with Brett from years ago. When the display appeared on the mobile X-ray machine, it confirmed the diagnosis. This was a pneumothorax. The needle from the central line insertion had pierced the pleura. I rapidly gathered the equipment needed and then inserted a chest drain. Irene's parameters soon improved. Both her oxygen saturations and her blood pressure had normalised rapidly.

As Hannah and I sat down a couple of hours later to debrief, I could see how devastated she was. I could imagine that same dreaded word appearing in her mind – as it did for me years ago – INCOMPETENT. I tried my best to convince her that her technique was sound, that this was a recognised complication, and that it happens to the best intensivists. She apologised profusely, but I insisted it was not necessary. I failed to realise that performing well and teaching well were two different skillsets. While I had the competence and confidence to insert central lines myself, and was fortunate enough to have very few complications, I had not developed the ability to supervise them competently. Unlike the adage, I had not smoothly sailed through seeing, doing, and teaching. I was, in fact, the incompetent party in this episode.

As I cycled home that evening, I wondered to myself. Should I have let Hannah continue when I noticed the depth of her needle? I was convinced this would not have made a difference, since if she had already pierced the pleura, then it was unlikely she would cause further lung damage by continuing with the insertion. Yet, I could not ignore the complication Irene had suffered because of Hannah's learning experience. The fundamental oath to "do no harm" seemed incongruent to the etymological identity of the "doctor". If being a doctor is to teach, and to learn procedures necessitates making mistakes which are sometimes harmful, how can one avoid being complicit in the violation of one's oath?

Perhaps the analogy of a string instrument like the double bass is again useful. The strings are held in tension at both ends of the instrument, and it is through this tension that music is created. If tension is released at either end, the string fails to serve its purpose altogether. Consequently, if tension is too great, strings may snap (admittedly more common for violins than the thick strings of the double bass).

The advent of simulation training within medicine has bridged some of the tensions between these two requirements of being a doctor. Simulation provides a safe environment to practise a skill without complications to patients. It allows for the repetition of procedures within a short space of time to build muscle memory. Some forms of simulation facilitate analyses and improvement of teamwork. Yet, simulation is not always an ideal substitute for real-life experiences. Our procedural simulators are sometimes unable to adequately replicate the feel of real human tissue, nor account for the differences in individual anatomy, nor the frequently suboptimal clinical circumstances we find ourselves in while needing to perform a procedure. Simulation is often costly, if not for the actual simulator, then for the time it takes the doctor away from clinical work. This is especially the case for a healthcare system which is obsessed with frugality and efficiency. Time spent practising is sometimes considered less important than performing clinical duties, since on-call rotas must be filled, and patients must be seen. So, the cost of safer performance and fewer complications is burdened on the trainees, who spend countless hours and inordinate amounts of money to be the best they can be.[13]

The thought that a doctor might be expected to perform a procedure only after seeing it a couple of times seems scary. However, one must not forget the years of study and practice that allow us to apply transferrable skills and knowledge to unfamiliar territories. Anatomy is taught in medical school and continues to feature heavily in many postgraduate exams. As a roadmap of the body, we know key areas relevant to our practice. Procedures like central lines and drains, as well as ultrasound-guided nerve blocks, utilise similar procedural principles.

The Seldinger technique, pioneered by the Swedish radiologist Sven-Ivar Seldinger in 1952, transformed the way doctors gained access to blood vessels. Threading a wire into a hollow needle after puncturing the desired vessel or cavity allowed the practitioner to maintain access while exchanging the small needle for larger drains or catheters. This dramatically reduced the complication rates of the then-widely practised method of using large, sharp trocars to pierce body cavities. With the Seldinger technique, practitioners could access smaller vessels, and drain various cavities. This forms the basis for many of our procedures and thus provides a firm anchor even in uncharted waters.

They say that in jazz, "playing a wrong note once is a mistake, but playing it twice is jammin'". I found this encouraging when I was learning how to play jazz as a teenager. It gave me an excuse for making mistakes during improvisation. It provided the freedom of artistic expression without being judged for playing the "wrong notes". This, in turn, honed my skills in improvisation and encouraged me to push my skills further. Without a doubt, mistakes are not merely inconveniences in learning skills. They are necessary. Not mistakes in themselves,

---

[13] In 2017, the Association of Surgeons in Training estimated that each trainee spent close to £20,000 of their own money on courses, conferences, and exams throughout their surgical training. O'Callaghan J, Mohan HM, Sharrock A, Gokani V, Fitzgerald JE, Williams AP, *et al*. Cross-sectional study of the financial cost of training to the surgical trainee in the UK and Ireland. BMJ Open. 2017;7(11):e018086.

though. Of far greater importance is the reaction to a mistake. The elite athlete tries harder after a stumble. The musician hones his skill from hours of practice and countless attempts. Likewise, doctors must continue to be allowed to learn from their mistakes without the spectre of litigation or embarrassment constantly hanging over their heads.

Neurosurgeon Dr Henry Marsh, in his memoir *Do No Harm*, writes about the emotional turmoil he experienced having to face a patient with an operative complication which resulted in permanent injury. He had allowed his junior surgeon to operate, but a mistake had been made, and a major nerve had been cut. The mistake colours his life, his future decisions, and the way he relegates control to his juniors. Like in the Thai horror film *Shutter*, Marsh's demons weigh heavily on his shoulders. So, too, do my mistakes burden my conscience, no doubt altering the way I relate to supervision as I progress through the training programme.

Today, I still get nervous at crucial points while supervising juniors for procedures. Yet in these moments, courage is demonstrated not just in continuing to allow juniors to learn, but also in taking overall responsibility for potential complications. And critically ill patients need such courage. Courage that is vital when "refer to critical care" comes at the end of many treatment algorithms. It is essential when we offer patients life-sustaining treatment, knowing that the cost of survivorship is heavy. It is crucial when we decline life support for patients who would not benefit.

Just as surgeons make ever braver decisions to operate on ever frailer patients, courage thus extends beyond practical skills to our decision-making. We know not who will survive or, indeed, who may benefit from intensive care. Yet, we are expected to possess the courage to make such decisions, even if we are proven wrong sometimes. When life is at stake all the time, our hearts must continue to become those of lions.

After Hannah's case, I pay far more attention to the needle depth when supervising central line insertions. But this is just one example of the need to be eagle-eyed. It is sharpness that identifies mistakes before they occur, from the minor complication of invasive procedures to the potentially fatal drug error. Each procedure I supervise, and each ward round I lead, I gain further experience in developing precision and acuity. Finally, I learnt gentleness from Chris's handling of my mistake. His skill and graciousness saved Brett from further complications and me from wallowing in self-pity. So, while I still have not figured out the best way to balance the need to *see one, do one, teach one* with the oath to *do no harm*, I continue to hope that my experiences have propelled me closer to the goal of the *eyes of an eagle, heart of a lion and hands of a lady*.

> *"It's not the note you play that's the wrong note – it's the note you play afterwards that makes it right or wrong." - Miles Davis*

9. AAA:
Abdominal Aortic Aneurysm

"Only magic can cure tumours of the vessels (referring to aneurysms)"
- Ebers papyrus (ca. 1550 BCE)

Acquit

I was a foundation doctor working in A&E when I saw
Marcus. He had been brought in by ambulance one night after
severe back pain. He had been put into the resuscitation bay
(Resus) by the paramedics not just due to a racing heart
(tachycardia) but because he just "looked like crap". I had only
worked a few shifts in Resus prior to this. I was young and
excited, ready to test my diagnostic skills, and keen for action.
While back pain seemed an unlikely reason to be put into Resus,
the paramedics' sixth sense for critical illness was not to be
ignored. It was a busy night for the them, and I got a very brief
handover before they shot off to their next call.

"Marcus Taylor, 67-year-old, complaining of sudden onset
back pain this evening. No trauma. Past medical history of
hypertension. Difficult to get a reliable blood pressure in the
ambulance, but he doesn't look right, doc."

While I got the handover, senior nurse Pam attached
monitoring. First the blood pressure cuff, followed by the ECG
electrodes, and then the pulse oximeter. After the handover, I
attempted a history but soon realised Marcus was too drowsy to
answer my questions. So, I went through a general examination
instead, following the ABCDE approach that was drilled into me
at medical school.

Airway: Seemed patent. No snoring or obstructive noises.

Breathing: A high respiratory rate of 30, but he did not look like
he was struggling to breathe. His chest had no obvious injuries,
and expansion was good, with normal breath sounds. This was
reassuring.

Circulation: Tachycardia, as noted by the monitor, at 120 beats
per minute, but normal heart sounds. He looked peripherally

shut down. His hands and feet were cold. His skin was grey. I took a mental note of these adverse signs and sped up.

Disability: He moaned when I called his name but obeyed my commands to squeeze my fingers. His eyes were shut, but I wasn't sure if this was due to pain. When I pulled them open, the pupils were both equal and reactive.

Exposure: His abdomen felt tense, and I noted the grimaces with each palpation. Indeed, this was no ordinary back pain.

I glanced to the monitor again, after the beep that signalled a blood pressure reading: 76/40.

Marcus was in shock. His blood pressure was dangerously low, explaining his low level of consciousness and dreadful appearance. If nothing was done, a cardiac arrest would ensue very rapidly. My jaw tightened as I realised the severity of the situation. Suddenly, everything sped up a notch.

"Bag of Hartmann's please, Pam", I asked as I wrapped a tourniquet around Marcus' arm. Despite the low blood pressure, his veins were visible, and as soon as a large cannula went in, blood was drawn and sent to the lab. By this time, Pam had set up the bag of fluid, so I connected it and let it run freely. Each drop was buying time as I searched for a diagnosis.

In my mind, the usual differentials of kidney stones or mechanical back pain were replaced by a single important diagnosis. As I wheeled the ultrasound machine from the next bay and popped the probe onto the middle of his abdomen, my fears were confirmed. There it was: the layers of blood from the ruptured abdominal aortic aneurysm resembling an onion, beautiful but deadly. The main blood vessel, the aorta, which serves as a conduit from the heart to the rest of the body, had dilated and then burst. If not for the intrinsic clotting abilities of the body, Marcus would exsanguinate within minutes. The thin and fragile clots that formed around the aorta gave it the onion-like appearance on the ultrasound.

"Shit!" I exclaimed out loud, much to Pam's surprise, who looked at the screen curiously and then at me. "Ruptured AAA," I said. Immediately, she went to get help. Within two minutes, a consultant and another senior doctor arrived, took one look at the image on the screen, and said to me, "Good spot, Mark. Can you give the vascular centre a call to transfer him over. We will help with the resuscitation here."

I left Resus and picked up the closest phone.

"Switchboard."

"Hello, may I please speak to the vascular registrar on call at the QE hospital?"

"Hold on," said the switchboard operator. Some inappropriately serene and non-committal music played as I waited.

"Hi, Ahmed, vascular reg[istrar]."

"Hi, I'm Mark, one of the doctors calling from A&E in Queen Victoria Hospital. Can I refer a patient, please?"

"Yes, go ahead."

"I've got a 67-year-old gentleman with known hypertension who has come in with severe back pain. We've done an ultrasound scan: he has a ruptured triple-A. He is in shock with blood pressure of 76/40 and heart rate of 120."

"Oh ok, who has done the scan?"

"Me"

"What grade are you?"

"FY2," I admitted, knowing where this was going. He would doubt my findings and ask for a senior review. He would try to make us obtain CT evidence, but this would delay the transfer. We had no vascular expertise in that district general hospital, and Marcus needed an emergency transfer to stand any chance of survival.

"Has your registrar or consultant seen him?" he sceptically asked.

"Yes, they are with the patient at the moment but asked me to call you."

"Can you get a CT scan to confirm the findings?"

"No, I think he is too unstable."

"But we need to know where exactly the AAA is."

"Yes, but if we put him through the scanner, he will die. You need to take this man to your hospital now! You can scan him there if you want. I'm not putting him through a scanner here." I almost shouted. Marcus would die without a transfer and an operation, but here I was, wasting time arguing with a registrar doubting my findings. I knew he couldn't see it, but my hands continued to gesticulate wildly while the phone was held against my shoulder, as if it would get my point across more effectively.

"How can we be sure it really is a AAA then without the CT?" he asked.

"We have seen it on ultrasound, and my consultant has confirmed my findings. This man does not need a CT scan now; he needs to go to a vascular centre."

The line went silent for a few seconds. Ahmed was taken aback by my boldness, but he must have mumbled a very soft affirmative. I next remembered hanging up, running to the coordinator to order an ambulance, and then back to Resus to tell my consultant.

Marcus' blood pressure was marginally better, at 88/49. His heart rate had settled to 105 with the fluid that was infused. Emergency blood had been started, and the anaesthetists were called to help with the transfer. My consultant, Chris, then left me with the registrar to continue the resuscitation while he went out of Resus to look for Marcus' wife. I saw them walk into the relatives' room.

I was too junior, at that stage, to be handling conversations like that, but I knew full well what information Chris would have covered. The shock was written on her face as they both entered Resus a few minutes later. Due to the need for an urgent transfer, Marcus' wife had little time to process the information. Instead of a Kubler-Ross progression through the stages of grief,[14] she was hit with a truckload of dire news and then sent to be with her husband for the transfer. I knew it was likely the last time she would see him, and I busied myself with the last preparations. Somehow, I tried to avoid making too much eye contact with her, cowardly fearing that somehow my eyes would

---

[14] Elizabeth Kubler-Ross was famous for publishing her stages of grief. In her work, she noted that most people go through five predictable stages when given bad news: denial, anger, bargaining, depression, and acceptance. Today, we know that not everyone goes through all five stages, the duration spent in each stage is unpredictable, and they do not progress in a linear fashion. Some people may flit from one stage to another, while others may skip a stage. Some people quickly ran through the stages to acceptance, while others get stuck at depression for years. Grief is thus a very individual process, and while the five stages provide some framework with which to understand emotional processing, it is not a rulebook.

give away my fear for Marcus' life. She knew. I saw it in the quivering lip, in the tears which welled up at the corner of her eye, in the hand which grasped on tightly to his.

Soon, the paramedics arrived, and they were gone.

I sat in the doctors' office just before the end of my shift. My adrenaline-fuelled trembling had finally started to subside, and my heart slowed down. After all, I was a new doctor, just over a year after qualifying from medical school. This was a classic surgical emergency I learnt about in medical school, but despite the theoretical knowledge, I was unprepared for the speed of the resuscitation, as well as the discomfort it stirred within me. I let out a big sigh of relief, glad that Marcus was heading to the vascular centre.

The manic rush of resuscitation, the frustration of an argument with the vascular registrar and the uncertainty of Marcus' survival finally manifested in the tears which welled up in my eyes. My shoulders slumped as I slouched back into the office chair and stared into the computer, unable to register what was on the screen. In my head, my mind replayed the images of the critically ill Marcus and the bomb that exploded within his abdomen. I imagined the state in which he would arrive at the vascular centre – shocked, likely semi-comatose, in pain, or worse, dead. I hoped I had done well, but more than that, I hoped that our resuscitative efforts were sufficient to support his life until emergency surgery. I hoped that my argument with the vascular registrar bought Marcus the time he needed to get to theatre. I hoped that we had given Marcus the best chance we could.

My consultant – sat beside me – noted my apparent despair, and simply said, "You did well, Mark. That was one of the fastest resuscitation and transfers for an AAA I've been involved in. Go get a cup of tea before handover."

For weeks, I wondered how Marcus fared, armed with the knowledge that most patients with ruptured AAAs die. While the compliment may have galvanised my training experience, it provided none of the certainty of results. The lack of centralised health information systems and the busyness of A&E rotas meant I was unable to find out if Marcus was even alive.

Two months later, I had rotated to a general surgical job in the same hospital. On day two of this rotation, during the ward round one morning, a familiar name appeared on the list. There, written on the handover:

Patient	Clinical Details	Past Medical History	Progress	Jobs
Marcus Taylor 22/02/1950	Repatriated from QE. Ruptured AAA repair	Hypertension	Doing well	Recheck renal function

An Emmaus moment for me; the recognition of his name warmed my heart. No longer uncertain of his fate, I had witnessed Marcus' revival from the near-death experience in A&E two months prior. He had had his ruptured aneurysm repaired and was on the ICU for a few weeks, with delirium and kidney failure, but managed to wean off renal replacement therapy. After he was stable, he was transferred back to the local hospital.

As the most junior member of the team, I did not say anything to Marcus during the ward round. But in the afternoon, I returned.

"Hi Marcus, my name is Mark. You met me this morning, but you might not remember I actually saw you in A&E when you first came in a couple of months ago."

"Did you? I don't remember," he said, with a mildly puzzled look on his face.

"Don't worry. You were rather drowsy then, so it's unsurprising you don't remember. Well, you were very sick and I'm really glad you managed to get the operation and have recovered so well."

"Oh. Sorry. I really don't recall."

My vanity wanted him to remember our efforts. My ego wanted him to know how I diagnosed his AAA. My pride wanted him to understand how I punched above my weight and won the argument with the vascular registrar. But perhaps it was a blessing that Marcus did not remember the numerous members of staff fighting on his behalf in that A&E. The explanation for amnesia was physiological. Poor circulation meant that Marcus' brain was poorly perfused and incapable of generating a clear memory of the event. But the amnesia was also meta-physiological, perhaps divinely, for the scene of critical illness resembled a battlefield more than what Anatole Broyard called a "parade ground".

He was spared the memory. I was spared the self-importance.

Pam had called for help. Chris had directed the resuscitation and communicated with Marcus' wife. Ahmed had operated on him.

I was but a pawn in his victory.

"Don't worry. It doesn't matter. It's good to see you so well," I said, as I smiled and then took my leave.

"Thank you," he said with a slightly perplexed look on his face.

Marcus was very lucky. Most others are not.

Asunder

I was an anaesthetics and intensive care registrar when I saw Janice in A&E, who had also suffered a ruptured AAA. She was less drowsy than Marcus and had arrived at the hospital with her son, James. Unsurprisingly, Janice complained of sudden onset abdominal pain. When the A&E doctor put an ultrasound probe on her abdomen, he immediately recognised the distinctive layered appearance of a ruptured AAA. In many aspects, her vital observations were less adverse than with Marcus: her blood pressure was higher, she was more awake, and more importantly, her skin colour was pink, unlike the pale, grey hue of near-death.

I spoke to Janice and her son James about how ill she was, about how she needed the operation, but also about how she was likely to die despite our best efforts. I did most of the talking, aware of the speechlessness which would inevitably follow such an awful diagnosis. After all, my experience with Marcus cycled over and over in my head over the years, and through it, I had prepared myself for a conversation like this.

As expected, both Janice and James cried. I emphasised the importance of the operation, but I also told them the truth – that most patients with ruptured AAAs do not survive. I thought it was better to prepare them for the worst and have a pleasant surprise than vice versa.

Normally, we would not have allowed visitors to the theatre complex, but we allowed James to accompany Janice all the way to the anaesthetic room, an attempt to temper the harsh reality of an almost certain, sudden, and horrific death. He was mostly silent as he held his mother's hand. Theatre was ready, and the theatre practitioner, Andy, and I began pushing the bed swiftly around the corridors, into the lift and down into the catacombs of the theatre department, where my other anaesthetic colleagues were waiting, drugs and equipment all prepared.

As we wheeled the bed, I explained to Janice and James what would happen in theatre, telling them about the process of anaesthesia and the need for the surgeons to be ready to cut immediately after induction of anaesthesia. Again, I stressed the severity of the situation but emphasised it was impossible to tell who would do well. Secretly, I was hopeful: Janice was relatively young with fewer comorbidities than many other patients. She had presented to a hospital with emergency vascular services. She was less shocked than patients like Marcus. But I suspected that my constant frown, my furrowed brows, and my clenched teeth gave away my nervousness.

As we approached the emergency theatre, we stopped for a moment so that James could say goodbye. He held onto Janice's hand, kissed her forehead, and said softly, "I love you Mum." Then she was in theatre, fear evident as I looked her in the eye. The surgeons cleaned and prepared the abdomen before we anaesthetised Janice. She looked at me, clearly afraid that the surgeons were about to start without anaesthesia. I reassured her this would not happen, but it was done to minimise the time between anaesthesia and incision. As I held the mask to her face, I managed a practised smile as I muttered, "We'll take good care of you, Janice."

As soon as the drugs entered Janice's circulation, her blood pressure plummeted. The tamponade effect of her muscles was abolished by anaesthesia and surgical incision. The emergency adrenaline we prepared was injected, a drug usually only used for cardiac arrests. The blood pressure fell further. Bags of blood, plasma and platelets were forced into Janice by pressure infusers, but her heart pumped them back out through the aorta right into the surgical field. The surgeon, having performed a midline incision, was retracting the rest of the abdominal organs to get access to the aorta for clamping. This part of the procedure, unchanged from original descriptions by Antyllus in c.400 BCE,[15] took an unusually long time. As the minutes ticked, the furrows on the surgeon's brow deepened. I glanced over the drapes in between the adrenaline and the next bag of blood and caught the shakes of the surgeon's head and the mumbled curses, followed by trying several alternative instruments.

"How is it coming along on your end? She's needing a lot of blood and adrenaline for that blood pressure," the anaesthetic consultant said to the surgeon.

"There are too many adhesions. I just can't get my clamp on effectively," came the exasperated reply.

Unable to get into position to clamp the aorta, the bleeding would not stop. The blood products, the multiple drugs used to optimise coagulation, the adrenaline, the rapid attempts of dividing adhesions. None were sufficient, and eventually, we were all utterly defeated.

"I still can't get control. I think it's time to stop," said the surgeon.

"I agree. Anyone have any objections?" said the anaesthetic consultant while looking around. She could see the fatigue on everyone's faces. Shakes of heads all round.

We then stood and watched as the blood pressure dropped, the ECG signals dwindled, and the tone of the oxygen saturations descended, until Janice's life was made asunder. Time of death: 0256 hours.

"We'll take good care of you, Janice" were the last words she heard. Presumption, confidence, or false belief, or perhaps comfort, compassion or dedication. I wrestled with these words for days. If it was impossible to predict mortality, why the false reassurance? If we were unable to ensure success, why the

---

[15] Desperate attempts of treating AAAs from the late 1800s involved injecting foreign material into the aneurysmal sac to promote thrombosis and coagulation. This, in theory, would reduce the shear force and turbulence of blood on the aneurysmal walls, thus encouraging a more laminar flow through the pre-morbid orifice. However, these techniques were met with almost no curative success, despite symptomatic relief in some patients.

seemingly half-hearted mutterings? What else were we to say? How else were we to approach such situations?

No, good medical care does not solely depend on mortality rates or lives saved. After all, the early Byzantine Christians, in contrast to the prevailing practice of physicians of leaving terminally ill patients, stood by their convictions to care for the sick and dying. While Greek physicians then were abandoning even their emperors, Christians were caring for sufferers of the plague, evicted from their households for fear of contamination and transmission.[16,17] It was this commitment to the sick and poor that transformed the practice of Western medicine, re-aligning it with the earlier Hippocratic suggestion, "Where there is love for man, there is also love for the art of medicine." For this is love which endures, which waits, which cries, and which refuses to be defeated in the face of death. Yes, "good" was no spectacular rescue, no fantastic miracle, no superhuman act.

Despite centuries of medical advances, the ability to manipulate physiology, masterful surgical expertise and seamless teamwork, Janice succumbed to the beast which had grown in her belly. Yet, "good" was precisely compassionate and committed care, adherence to the ancient Egyptian advice on the treatment of ruptured aneurysms, "Do not abandon them."[18]

"We took good care of you, Janice."

Acumen

Neither Marcus nor Janice had knowledge of their abdominal aortic aneurysms before their emergency presentations to hospital. Fortunately, the AAA screening programme in England was launched in 2013. Thanks to the screening of high-risk populations and regular surveillance, many people can undertake AAA repairs before they rupture. These procedures carry far lower mortality rates than undertaking a repair once it ruptures.

---

[16] Lascaratos J, Poulakou-Rebelakou E, Marketos S. Abandonment of terminally ill patients in the Byzantine era. An ancient tradition? J Med Ethics. 1999;25(3):254-8.

[17] Aitken JT, Aitken JT, Fuller HWC, Johnson D, Christian Medical F. The Influence of Christians in medicine1984.

[18] Cooley DA. A Brief History of Aortic Aneurysm Surgery. Aorta (Stamford). 2013;1(1):1-3.

The decision to operate may be straightforward for some patients, but for the very elderly or highly co-morbid, models and calculations sometimes do not adequately capture the nuances of quality of life, complications, or expected functional recovery. This was the case with Dennis.

Dennis was 84 years old. He was unable to give me a history. When I saw him in A&E, he was just as shocked as Marcus was. Drowsy, confused, and in pain, the only information I had were his worrying vital signs, the result of a bedside ultrasound that demonstrated a ruptured AAA, and a plastic bag containing about ten different medications. He looked frail, but the ambulance crew had told me that he was independent with his daily activities, and a keen gardener.

Should Dennis be resuscitated? At 84, with several comorbidities, would he even survive such a major operation? Should he even be offered it? What would his quality of life be afterwards? Would it be better to palliate him and prioritise comfort? What were his best interests? What would *he* want? These were the questions which ran through my mind as I weighed up the options. These questions plague every intensivist when seeing patients who are unable to furnish us with coherent histories. Unlike many specialities, which rely on patient history for diagnosis and the subsequent discussion of management options, intensive care medicine sometimes necessitates a strongly paternalistic approach until patients' wishes are known or communicated.

So, I spent the next hour resuscitating Dennis and contacting the nearest vascular centre for transfer. Fluids were needed for his blood pressure, yet not too much as to shear the clot which had invariably formed around the aorta. Analgesia was provided for the pain, alongside supplemental oxygen for maximal delivery to organs and tissues. Dennis started waking up when his blood pressure was high enough to perfuse his brain, but then just as quickly slumped back into his stuporous state before a small dose of vasopressor enabled another question or two. I was just about to order a CT scan when a nurse asked if his wife could come in. I had forgotten about that. I said yes and prepared myself for a difficult discussion, like the one I had with Janice's son.

"Your husband has an aortic aneurysm. The big blood vessel running down the middle of his abdomen has burst and is leaking blood into the tummy. He is critically ill. I was just about to call the vascular surgeons to see if we can get him transferred for an emergency operation," I said.

"I know. He doesn't want it operating on," she said calmly.

"What?" I recoiled.

"We know he has a triple-A. It was diagnosed last year, but we had discussions with the consultant and decided that he did not want an operation for it."

I did not expect this answer. My previous experiences with ruptured AAAs were unanimously dramatic, hasty, and stressful. Those conversations were practised, and while the information was unpleasant, I was used to it. This time, faced with an unexpected advanced care decision, I needed a few seconds to reorganise my strategies.

"Oh… ok, you do know he will die without the operation," I checked.

"Yes, we know."

Dennis was more awake by this time and corroborated the information and conversation I just had with his wife. He felt little pain by now, thanks to the morphine. I felt relieved, not so much that I escaped a difficult discussion, but because Dennis and his wife had known about his diagnosis, had discussed its implications, and had made an informed, measured and personal decision about management.

Instead of a rushed conversation about emergency surgery and emphasis on the likelihood of intraoperative death, I was able to explore their priorities on analgesia and anxiolysis, on mental and spiritual health, on options of place of death.

There was no anguish of Gethsemane, no Homeric chaos.

Instead, it was calm, collected, and dignified, just like how most would prefer terminal illness to be. Indeed, there was a serenity about Dennis – one who had seen the face of angels, had sung the songs of victory, and had won the battle even before it began. As I held his hand before he left A&E, I felt no fear of his demise. In his eyes, I realised the power of the lyrics, *"No guilt in life, no fear in death…"* by Stuart Townend.

Dennis' knowledge of his "triple A" meant a controlled, dignified death, rather than the triple shock of diagnosis, prognosis, and *mortis*. It meant a gradual ascent into heaven rather than an abrupt plunge into the abyss. A diminuendo into silence instead of a sforzando exit. I admired Dennis – admired his courage, his dignity, his genius.

"I want to go when I want. It is tasteless to prolong life artificially."
- Albert Einstein, on refusing repeat surgery after a ruptured AAA.

Postscript

During my anaesthetic training, I remember being involved in my first elective, open AAA repair. Before this, I had only been involved in emergency ruptured AAA repairs. I was nervous. I thought that it would be as chaotic as the previously described cases. When I asked my consultant if I should prepare emergency adrenaline, he laughed at me.

I had imagined wild cardiovascular changes and instability because that was what happened with the emergency cases. But instead, the scene was far more controlled. The patient entered the operating theatre in a stable physiological position. She was not in excruciating pain. She was not rushed into making decisions. She had had several conversations with the surgeon and anaesthetist to ensure she understood the severity of the condition, the risks of the procedure, and the potential complications. For her, as in many elective AAA repairs, the procedure progressed at a steady pace. The team knew what to expect, and although we anaesthetists learn about the severe cardiovascular sequelae of certain steps of the operation, these are often far less profound than we imagine. The survival rate is far higher than for ruptured AAA repairs. It was, in all respects, a far more satisfactory journey compared to what Marcus and Janice went through.

Marcus never remembered his ordeal but would clearly have died without the operation. Janice never remembered her ordeal but died with us trying to save her life. Under anaesthesia, she felt no pain, had no awareness, and slipped, without fanfare, into the realms of the gods. This, one might argue, may constitute a "good death". But what of her son, James, who experienced the trauma of the sudden demise of his mother, of being unable to be there when she died, of being told by the doctors, "We tried our best, but…"? Surely his scars will stay with him for years to come?

The AAA screening programme has made elective AAA repairs more common. As a result, patients with ruptured AAAs are far more uncommon these days than they used to be. Yet, the occasional patient slips through the net. Generally, these are young men who have not yet been screened. Or they are women, who are currently not covered by the screening programme since they rarely develop AAAs.

As I reflect on the extremes of these cases, I ponder what Nortin Hadler described as the four pillars of octogenarians: self-actualisation, interaction, independence, and comfort.[19] This was a play on the more widely known four pillars of medical ethics: autonomy, beneficence, non-maleficence, and justice. We learnt these four pillars in medical school. We are tested on them in postgraduate exams. These pillars form fundamental foci when trying to make difficult decisions. For example, we decided for Marcus that an operation was to his benefit, and by doing so, we would not cause him further harm (since he would die without one). He was unable to make an autonomous decision due to his condition, and so, using the pillars, we transferred him to the vascular centre. Dennis, by comparison, made an advanced autonomous decision not to operate on his AAA. This overrode my initial plan for surgery, based on beneficence and non-maleficence.

Hadler's twist to the four pillars shifts the focus from an assumed priority of preservation of life to one that is equally just and beneficial – maintenance of quality of life – and facilitation of a dignified death. For me, Dennis' knowledge of his terminal illness allowed him the independence and self-actualisation to plan his own death. It facilitated meaningful interaction, not just with healthcare providers but also with his loved ones. Above all, it afforded the comfort of expectation, adaptation, and closure. To me, there was little argument that his journey constituted a "good death".

---

[19] Hadler N. The last well person. Quebec: McGill-Queen's University Press; 2004.

10. Tiny Oars

I wept. I wept at the morning handover. I broke down in front of my colleagues. I sobbed like a baby, had it not been dead. I wept like a grieving mother, had she not been dead too. Two deaths in one night.

The obstetric consultant stood outside theatre and cried. The senior midwife walked, in a daze, back to her station. I glanced at two other midwives crying in the corner, held in each other's arms. I quickly walked past, as the tears welled up, into the anaesthetic office, and cried. My colleague, Bibha, who had been working with me through the night, slumped into her chair, silent. It would be a few hours yet before she cried. The day-shift anaesthetists, Horace and Mo, sat in silence opposite us in the crammed anaesthetic office. Horace put his hand on my shoulder, and I cried even harder. Drips soon became streams of tears.

I saw Blessing in A&E's Resus Bay in the middle of the night. She did not see me. She was too drowsy. It was a busy night for me as the on-call anaesthetist for maternity. In between the emergency Caesarian sections and the multiple calls for epidurals, I overheard the midwife-in-charge mumble a single phrase which immediately stopped me in my tracks,

"Hold on, Mark, there might be a peri-mortem section."[20]

The details were sketchy, so I followed midwife Katie out of the labour ward down to A&E, where she was heading to join the obstetric consultant, Mr Ali. As we arrived in A&E, I got a brief handover,

"25-year-old lady, 28 weeks [pregnant]. Sudden onset abdominal pain. She's been shocked and barely responsive since she arrived. This is her gas. She's acidotic. Her haemoglobin has dropped from 90 to 67. Surgeons were also called, and a CT scan has been ordered but they can't detect a foetal heartbeat now."

---

[20] This catastrophic emergency involves performing a Caesarian section immediately when the life of the mother is in danger (peri-mortem), prioritising the life of the mother over the foetus which might be alive or dead.

I let myself past the drawn curtains into the small cubicle. Mr Ali held the curved abdominal ultrasound probe on Blessing's tummy. I helped him adjust the depth and brightness of the image on the machine. We saw the foetus. The miniature human, almost fully formed, with brain, limbs, and organs. But no foetal heartbeat. It was dead. He scanned further down; the placenta looked large and irregular. It just did not look right. We needed to go to theatre, both to find the source of the bleeding as well as to stop the dead foetus causing further bleeding problems.

"Let me do a quick assessment now," I said. Several questions needed answering immediately: was it safe to transfer Blessing up to theatre? Did we have to perform the C-section imminently? If Blessing's life was immediately threatened, we would have had no choice but to do it in A&E. Fortunately, with the fluids she had been given, her blood pressure was respectable.

We saw a window of opportunity and took it.

I called my consultant and the other anaesthetic registrar on-call for help. We sent blood for transfusion directly up to theatre from the lab. En route, we passed Blessing's husband, who was waiting in the corridor. Mr Ali told him briefly that she was bleeding and she needed to go to theatre to stop it. He kissed her on the forehead. A last kiss, although we did not know it then. We carried on – we could still save her. The theatre team was already on standby. Within 20 minutes of assessment in A&E, we were up in theatre.

Blood was hung up and flowed into Blessing's veins. The obstetricians painted the abdomen brown with antiseptic. I whispered in Blessing's ear that we were about to send her off to sleep, and that we would try our best to take care of her. She probably wasn't conscious enough to hear. The obstetricians held the scalpel poised. We were ready. Drugs were given. Off to sleep. Intubated. Knife to skin. Blood in the abdomen. Gushing out. Uterus thin and pale. Knife to uterus. Foetus out. Placenta removed.

Blessing's pulse became slow and thready.

I gave adrenaline. My hand remained on her carotid pulse. More blood was suctioned out. A large clot was seen beside the uterus. I announced that her heart rate had become very slow.

The obstetricians said there was bleeding even behind the uterus. They... just... could... not... get... to... it.

Her heart stopped.

"I've lost her pulse. Cardiac arrest! Start CPR," I said to the junior obstetrician, Vicky. "Pull the buzzer", I said to the anaesthetic practitioner. "Get the defibrillator", I shouted at the runner. "We need more blood!" I huffed at anyone who would listen.

After several minutes of CPR, Blessing regained her pulse. By this time, a huge team had gathered in theatre: junior doctors, midwives, the medical registrar on-call. Most of them looked on in horror at the edges of the operating theatre. I sent them away; we had sufficient people. The medical registrar stayed to help consider all the options,

"Haemorrhage is the most likely cause," he said. Of course it was; I just needed the moral support.

More blood was already being forced in. Despite removing the foetus and placenta, the bleeding persisted. It was coming from somewhere else. The hospital's entire anaesthetic and intensive care teams had arrived to help. We inserted lines, managed the blood transfusions, monitored the situation, and administered strong drugs to maintain Blessing's blood pressure. Mr Ali closed the uterus. Vicky applied pressure on the upper abdomen to slow down the bleeding.

The general and vascular surgeon, Mr Koh, arrived. By now, blood filled the abdomen. It soaked through swab after swab. It covered the gloved hands of the obstetricians and surgeons. It dripped off the cover of the surgical drape, forming a crimson puddle at the end of the table. Empty bags of blood products, once yellow and red, were now transparent and laid in a corner. There were too many to count contemporaneously. We had to do it later.

Mr Koh removed all the swabs used to pack the abdomen and stop the bleeding. We expected this to result in another fall in blood pressure, so we anticipated and squeezed more blood in. We turned the infusions up. We ordered more blood. Our expectations were vastly exceeded, and as soon as the swabs were removed, she crashed. Faster and faster the blood flowed, like a burst dam, from her vessels straight into the reservoir of her abdomen. The exploration was futile; as each hand moved, they were like paddles against a rising crimson tide. Mr Koh had no choice. He gripped down on the aorta. This stopped all blood flow to the bottom half of the body. The bleeding slowed, but it was too late. We watched her blood pressure continue to disappear. She had another cardiac arrest.

CPR was restarted. Adrenaline was given. More blood products. The source of the bleeding was still unidentified. Hope was fading, but Mr Koh kept his grip firmly on the aorta, literally holding on for dear life. Jammed up right beside him, Vicky's bloodied hands pumped up and down on the chest. A couple of us continued to squeeze bag after bag of blood products into Blessing. The other surgeons continued to press on the abdomen, trying to soak up whatever bleeding they could. Over 30 minutes passed. She never regained her pulse. CPR was stopped.

The morning sun was rising, but the dawn was far from bright. The glaring operating lights remained on the lifeless corpse, but the entire theatre was overcome by darkness. Darkness which seeped out, like the blood still slowly staining the sheets, dripping from the body, stencilling the floor with countless crimson clog-prints from the numerous members of staff involved.

I was prepared for her death. I had four hours in theatre to be prepared. The two cardiac arrests weren't merely warning currents, they were riptides. The entire team was demolished, powerlessly crumbled by the force of exsanguination, ruthlessly swept away by the torrent of blood. I was prepared for her death. What I wasn't prepared for, was the conversation which ensued. But there was no conversation. In fact, our words were but a confirmation of the shadows which had already crept into the relatives' room at the far end of the corridor. Five of us walked into that room. Five sufficient pieces of information for the relatives to know that something was amiss. Chloe, the midwife who had spent the last few hours talking to and updating them, started the introductions.

"This is Jason, Blessing's husband," she gestured.

We didn't even get to say who we were. Jason stood up.

"Tell me. Is she alive?" he asked.

Mr Ali started, "I'm Mr Ali, the obstetric consultant. Sit down, let's talk."

"No, tell me she's alive."

"She has been bleeding badly."

"Please tell me she's alive…" Jason pleaded.

"No. I'm sorry, she has passed away."

"What?! No, no, no, no, no. This can't be true." The volume of his voice suddenly raised several notches.

"I'm really sorry, Jason. She has died."

Then, the shockwaves of horror shook the deepest recesses of all our beings. Jason's screams pierced deep into my heart. I had heard this scream before – the scream of a mother whose child had died in my hands years ago. We stood silent for what seemed an eternity, listening to the visceral, guttural, unrestrained call of sudden grief. Physically, I stood firm, but emotionally, I was completely overcome. There were no answers to their questions. No comfort for their exclamations. No reply to their cries. Instead, their streams of tears coalesced into raging rapids of sorrow, billowing and sweeping me along till my own steadfastness shifted. Cry after cry, like drops of Chinese water torture, steadily eroded my rigid professionalism.

There were no interludes to their cries, no break for the light of explanation to shine. We had to let them into the theatre to see the body. But that initial downpour merely presaged the inevitable storm of anguish. The entire theatre suite rumbled with their thunderous screams. And as the rains of grief fiercely battered the theatre, the waters of despair rose.

Wave after wave of agony pounded against my own firm foundations. I felt my own preparedness crumble under the onslaught of intense loss. For two further hours, it did not relent, and we all drowned in powerlessness. And when the cries subsided and the tears dried up, all that remained was a vast silence; the still sea that forever hid immeasurable depths of darkness. Our feeble clinical explanations, like tiny oars, did little to move the waters.

The numerous investigations and analyses dove deep but barely managed to capture the extent of the emotional ramifications, both for the clinical team and the family. Even the rays of understanding which eventually emerged from the postmortem examination merely penetrated the surface temporarily. Clinical answers, though enlightening, could not reverse the event. All we could do was acknowledge their grief and share their feelings of injustice.

We wept that morning. The family, the obstetric consultant, the midwives, the nurses, the theatre staff, and me. Crammed in the anaesthetics office, with my colleague's arm around my shoulders, I wept. I did not remember much of the drive home. My brain seemed still stuck underwater; the sounds of the theatre replayed in my ears, muffled. My vision, blurred by the tears I had shed, conveyed the red circles of speed limit signages, but all I could really see were the bags and bags of spent blood products, red-rimmed from the last bit of residue after administration, laid out on the floor in the corner of the theatre.

For a second, I noted everyone overtaking me; I was driving under 30 mph on a 50 mph road. The normal shuffle playlist of music was stopped. I could not bear to listen. Instead, Jason's screams echoed in my head, drowning out every other sound. The outline of the dead foetus on the ultrasound, curled up, partially formed, seared into my memory. I imagined my two daughters' faces superimposed on the outline. I imagined my own wife, just as young, just as beautiful, just as "fit and well". I imagined myself in Jason's shoes. I stopped. I had somehow safely reached my front gates, but I needed to get out to open them. I parked my car and plugged it in to be charged. I then walked through the door, hugged my wife, and wept.

I read to make sense of the injustice. I read about death: epidemiological reports, academic theses, poetry. I came across a poem by Norman MacGaig that struck a deep chord:

"There are fires to be suffered, the blaze of cruelty, the smoulder of inextinguishable longing, even the gentle candle flame of peace that burns too. I suffer them. I survive"

The use of fire as an allegory of grief and loss made an impression. The pain of a simple burn, and the subsequent throbbing felt during the recovery period seemed an adequate reminder of the event, even if not quite as acute. Yet the simplicity of that poem, for me, failed to capture the depth of the sorrow, and couldn't reflect the complexities of the multiple teams involved.

Fire suggested eventual extinguishment, which – at that time – I could not come to terms with. How could I ever forget such a case? How could the grief disappear? How could the sorrow eventually burn out? Instead, as I searched for another way to make sense of the tragedy, I drifted towards another unfathomable, untameable and unpredictable force of nature – water. From fluid dynamics, which reflected both exsanguination and lacrimation (crying), to storms and waves, which reflected emotional turmoil. From the peacefulness of still water to the darkness it conceals, water was the perfect allegory for my struggles surrounding this case. Water was both governable and unconquerable. It was both softly soothing yet overwhelmingly torturous. It was both transparent and impenetrable to light. Water could be many things to many people, but in this case, water seemed only sinister to me. Sinister and elusive, until one day, a song came on my playlist and sealed my meandering heart:

"How deep the father's love for us, How vast beyond all measure..."
- Stuart Townend

[Winner of the Society of Medical Writers' Autumn 2022 competition for non-fiction.]

11. An Ear on the Hive

"Blessed are you who have not seen, and yet have believed." John 20:29

I placed my stethoscope on the surface. A buzz. Not a contented one, but a moan. Perhaps. Or maybe not. I wasn't sure. I had little to compare with. This was unlike hearts or lungs, which my ears were far more accustomed to. It was the first honeybee swarm we collected. My wife and I had placed the bees into a freshly constructed wooden hive, but the bees did not like it. So they tried to abscond by leaving en masse.

Luckily, we had insurance in the form of a queen excluder over the entrance. But while, in principle, the small slits only allowed workers but not the larger queen to exit, the stampede caused by about 15,000 bees across the bottleneck of the entrance meant the unfortunate queen got stuck and died in the process (but we did not know it then). When the swarm eventually made their way back to the hive, having initially left their queen behind, they huddled on its surface.

After I finally discovered the dead queen, while removing the queen excluder to investigate further, the rest of the bees quickly made their way into the hive. I called my mentor. He suggested listening to the colony after a day. It is said that queenlessness may be identified by the collective moan of anarchy. So, I squatted behind the hive, placed the diaphragm of my Littmann Cardiology 3 stethoscope on the surface of the hive, and listened intently. But if one has no experience of community, how does one identify anarchy? It was only when we got our second swarm that we were able to compare the hum of a contented colony to the moan of a queenless one.

Similarly, clinical examination skills are honed throughout medical school and training. Clinical examination skills form a large part of undergraduate medical training. For exams, during the final few years of undergraduate training, we were judged on how well we performed the main examinations: cardiovascular (involving the heart and vessels), respiratory (involving lung pathologies), neurological (cranial nerves, upper limbs and lower limbs), and abdominal. The stethoscope was a key instrument for listening to heart, breath and bowel sounds. But to identify pathology, we needed to first familiarise ourselves with normality. So, my friends and I practised on each other. I remember spending hours after lectures and between clinical placements, sneaking into any spare room we could find in the university or hospital and repeating the process of conducting and presenting the examination.

Yet, abnormal sounds are sometimes subtle, and pathologies do not always neatly fit into clear categories. Take heart sounds, for example. We typically listen for the normal "lub-dub", which represents the closure of the four valves directing blood in a forward motion. A leaky valve (regurgitation) usually manifests as a "whoosh" of turbulence due to the backflow of blood when the heart contracts. Instead of a "lub-dub", mitral valve regurgitation may sound like a "whoosh-dub".

In contrast, there is the typical crescendo-decrescendo murmur of a narrowed valve (stenosis). The pressure needed to force blood through a smaller orifice builds up, delaying the onset of the sound, but due to the higher velocity of flow past the valve, the flow and the resultant turbulence cause a slow rise and fall compared to normal sounds. However, multiple valves can sometimes be affected, or single valves may manifest both regurgitation and stenosis, thus creating multiple sounds.

And then there are cardiac surgery patients. One can imagine – with the complexity of modern cardiac surgery – that identifying pathology purely based on heart sounds is extremely difficult. Enter heart ultrasound (echocardiography). Instead of relying on the interpretation of sounds, echocardiography uses ultrasound waves to create images of the heart, allowing us to essentially "look" into the heart in a real-time, dynamic fashion.

During my clinical examination for Membership of the Royal College of Physicians (otherwise known as MRCP PACES), I made my way through the cardiovascular examination. I saw the midline chest scar on my patient, signifying past cardiac surgery. There was a lack of a long scar on the leg, which normally indicates vein harvest for cardiac bypass surgery. So, I suspected he had had a valve/s replaced. I listened to his heart and indeed, there was a murmur which occurred during contraction of the ventricles (systole). This murmur was heard loudest over the aortic valve between the left ventricle and the main blood vessel supplying the body (the aorta). It was louder during exhalation and was not heard on the neck over the carotid arteries. Therefore, it was unlikely to be a narrowing of the aortic valve (aortic stenosis). There wasn't even the give-away click of a metallic prosthetic valve, either. Therefore, I concluded that the patient likely had valve replacement surgery and presented my findings as a "flow murmur characteristic of a tissue aortic valve replacement."

The examiner asked, "So, is that a pan-systolic murmur or an ejection systolic murmur?"[21]

"Neither. It is not louder in the mitral region, and there is no radiation to the axilla (armpit); therefore, it is not a pan-systolic murmur. There is no radiation to the carotids and no crescendo-decrescendo, so it is unlikely to be ejection systolic murmur of aortic stenosis. Therefore, it is a flow murmur, as is normal in a tissue aortic valve replacement. I would get an echocardiogram to confirm this." I replied confidently.

By this stage, I had already learnt how to perform focused echocardiography for diagnosis of gross cardiac problems.

"But does the valve replacement produce a pan-systolic or ejection systolic murmur?" the examiner pushed.

"Well, I would say neither, as the turbulence is merely due to a foreign valve, rather than a pathology of the valve. Besides, I would not diagnose a valvular lesion without an echocardiogram."

I stood my ground, and I failed that station.

To this day, I still do not know what the examiner wanted to hear, nor why he insisted that I commit to a particular murmur.

These days, valvular lesions are indeed diagnosed with an echocardiogram. The stethoscope may be useful for identifying abnormal heart sounds, but my ears are certainly not sharp enough to pick up subtle murmurs, especially since the complex patients I come across may have had all manner of cardiac operations, multiple valve pathologies, or are so critically ill that I wouldn't spend the time scrutinising the exact murmur.

---

[21] A pan-systolic murmur lasts throughout ventricular contraction and is characteristic of a regurgitant mitral valve. A crescendo-decrescendo ejection systolic murmur, on the other hand, is characteristic of aortic stenosis (and some other pathologies).

Instead, I chose to learn point-of-care ultrasonography and echocardiography early in my medical career. However, there were no trainers for this in the hospital where I worked. Instead, I had to contact mentors in a hospital an hour's drive away, do the paperwork allowing me to enter their hospital as visiting staff, and drive over on my days off until I was deemed competent. I am glad I persevered.

—————◆◆◆—————

"Mark, you're good at echo. Can you go see this patient for me, please?" my senior registrar, Tamara, said. "There's a 21-year-old gentleman on ward G2 who is being treated for endocarditis,[22] but they've called me because he has suddenly become extremely short of breath and needs 100% oxygen. Could you please go see what is happening?" "Sure," I replied, glad that my skills were being put to good use.

I was under a year into my anaesthetics training and was working in an intensive care unit in a large hospital. It was a night shift, at about 5 am in the morning. Before this, I had already worked as a clinical fellow (non-training job) in ICU for a year and had been performing point-of-care ultrasound then. Tamara knew I was enthusiastic about echo.

This time, I didn't even need to push the ultrasound machine all the way from the ICU to the other end of the hospital. The cardiology ward always had their own machine since echocardiograms were commonly done there. So, as I arrived and introduced myself to the nurse in charge, she directed me first to the echo machine, and then the patient.

The echo machine was a behemoth compared to the portable one we had in ICU. It was an old machine (the newer ones were reserved for the echocardiography department), and the off-white plastic body covered a full metal chassis protecting the computer hardware inside. As a result, it took considerable effort to push, despite the multi-directional wheels.

---

[22] Endocarditis describes an infection of the inner lining of the heart, frequently affecting the valves. Because the valves themselves do not receive any blood supply, and because the bacteria tend to form walled-off modules, endocarditis is difficult to treat even with antibiotics.

The console had a full keyboard with chunky keys, a tracking ball, and several knobs, unlike the newer portable ones with touchscreens. I pushed it to the patient's bedside and plugged it in immediately after I had introduced myself, knowing it would take at least five minutes to start up. Then I read the notes and took a history.

Sammy was only 21 years old. He was otherwise in good health but had spontaneously developed an infection of the inner lining of the heart, or endocarditis. The notes told me he had complained of some fevers and then chest pains. He had multiple blood cultures done to confirm the diagnosis, but before he could get a formal echocardiogram, he complained of sudden worsening chest pain and severe shortness of breath. The medical registrar was called in, but she very quickly realised he was struggling despite the oxygen provided. In fact, when I met him, he could only speak in single words. Through these "yes" and "no" replies, I was just about able to ascertain vague details about his admission and past medical history.

When I listened to Sammy's chest, there were crackles throughout his lung fields, indicating fluid within the lungs. The crackles were heard all the way to the top of his lungs, and that – coupled with low blood pressure and high heart rate – made me suspect left heart failure. But he was young; there was little reason for him to develop heart failure. He was not a heavy drinker, nor did he have any problems with his thyroid. Perhaps a viral infection of the heart muscle itself since he was admitted with an infection.

I put the ultrasound probe onto his chest, and thanks to his slim build, could immediately see the heart clearly. The left heart was severely dilated and could not pump efficiently. But the heart muscle looked normal, and all areas were contracting towards the middle as they should.

This was not viral myocarditis.

Instead, something did not look right. There was massive regurgitation of blood back from the left ventricle into the atrium. The mitral valve was completely incompetent! It was dramatically failing at its function to prevent the backflow of blood. I stared at it for another full minute, trying to figure out why this would be the case in a young man. Finally, I tried to explain my impression to Sammy.

"Normally, your mitral valve prevents any backflow of blood into your heart. But I think because of the endocarditis, one of the tendons, or heartstrings if you like, holding the valve in place has snapped, and this has caused the valve not to work as it should. Now, I'm not an expert at this scan, and I will make sure you get a formal scan to confirm what I suspect, but I think you've got what we call a flail posterior mitral leaflet. That is, one of the leaflets of the valve is flapping in the wind and unable to prevent backflow. This is why blood is congested back into your lungs and you are so breathless."

Sammy simply nodded.

I went on to tell him how we needed to contact the cardiothoracic unit at another hospital to get him transferred.

I wasn't entirely sure of the diagnosis, but I knew what I saw didn't look normal. I needed some confirmation, but Sammy needed urgent transfer to a cardiothoracic unit. I described my findings to my registrar, and we called the cardiothoracic unit together. In the meantime, Sammy was treated for acute heart failure, but this was likely a temporary fix. He needed the valve repaired or replaced.

The cardiothoracic unit agreed with our management plan, but also said they would discuss the case during the morning handover with a view to transferring him over that day. It was almost 7:30 am by this time, and the day shift was about to begin. The daytime consultant cardiologist had already been informed about my findings, along with the fact that I was not formally qualified to make such a diagnosis on the scan. He made his way into hospital earlier than normal to review the scan before we handed over the case.

As soon as I got home, I texted a day team colleague to ask about Sammy. The cardiologist had seen the videos I had saved on the machine and agreed completely with my diagnosis. They did not need to perform another formal scan. He had then also called the cardiothoracic unit to corroborate my findings. They transferred him across later that morning, but Sammy didn't go to surgery immediately. Because of the endocarditis, a valve replacement would carry a significant risk of re-infection, which would hamper his progress even further. So, with undying perseverance, Sammy tolerated treatment with potent antibiotics for several weeks.

Multiple drugs were required to maintain his blood pressure and control the fragile fluid balance in his body. Only after he completed the long course of antibiotics did the cardiothoracic team finally replace his valve. After that, Sammy made a swift recovery and – within another couple of weeks – went home and rapidly went back to university.

After that day, I somehow became an ultrasound "expert" in the eyes of the ICU team. I was soon asked to teach other registrars, and another consultant approached me to set up a training programme within the unit. By this time, I had already hung up my stethoscope. Who needed an outdated set of rubber tubes when one could see the structure of the heart directly? Why guess if a murmur was pan-systolic or ejection systolic, or bet on whether it originated from the mitral, aortic, tricuspid or pulmonary valve? What value was there in trying to determine if the crepitations heard on the lungs were because of infection or heart failure? No doubt this was a game changer in intensive care, so I thought. But I was soon to learn that even the most experienced eyes can be fooled.

<hr/>

"Much to learn you still have my young padawan." - Yoda. *Star Wars*

One day, we scanned Bob on the cardiothoracic critical care unit. Bob had had open heart and valve surgery the day prior. He was still on the ventilator and sedated. The drains which had been inserted into the site had minimal output, suggesting there was little bleeding. But over a few hours, he required more and more drug infusions to maintain his blood pressure. His heart rate rose, and his blood pressure slowly fell. We were concerned about a cardiac tamponade.[23]

---

[23] This occurs when blood or fluid collects in the sac surrounding the heart. Since the sac is rigid, the fluid could eventually impair the contraction of the heart as the pressure outside the heart exceeds the pressure generated inside. As this happens, less and less blood is pumped out towards the rest of the body and the organs suffer from lack of oxygen.

There were three junior doctors on that day who were accredited in focused echocardiography. We all scanned Bob's heart to look for fluid in the pericardium. We could not see any significant fluid, so we got an expert to corroborate our findings. Susan, the specialist echocardiography technician, came up to the ICU to perform a full scan. When she did, she concluded, just like us, that there was no significant fluid around the heart which would cause cardiac tamponade. However, by this time, Bob's blood pressure continued to fall, and he needed increasing amounts of drugs to maintain it. So, based on clinical suspicion, instead of a hard diagnosis, the consultants decided to take Bob back to theatre.

Within ten minutes of that decision, Bob was back in the operating theatre, where the surgeons re-opened his chest. There, behind the heart, hidden from the view of the echocardiogram we performed on the ICU itself, laid a large clot, a haematoma. This haematoma was compressing the right atrium, preventing blood from returning to the heart from the rest of the body. With insufficient blood returning, the heart was unable to pump it forward. Thus, Bob's blood pressure plummeted, and the heart raced in an attempt to pump more blood around the body. This was cardiac tamponade, indeed, but it was a localised tamponade rather than fluid accumulation around the entire sac. The surgeons rapidly removed the haematoma. After this, Bob's blood pressure recovered, and when he eventually made it back to the ICU again after closure of the chest, he very quickly improved and was extubated the day after. Within a few days, he was discharged to the ward and soon went home.

I felt terrible! I had steadily gained confidence in my ultrasound abilities. Just as I thought I had become good at focused echocardiography, medicine always finds a way to humble.

It is said within research circles, "The absence of evidence does not mean evidence of absence." Just because we failed to see fluid around the heart did not mean there wasn't any. It was merely hidden from our view. I was reminded of my inability to ever see 3-dimensional illusion pictures or stereograms. My father bought some when I was a child (like those sold by Magic

Eye), and I used to try for hours but could never see "beyond" the picture. I got frustrated and eventually gave up trying to see the 3D images.

Fortunately for Bob, the clinical acumen of the consultants mitigated the false confidence I had in the new skill I had acquired. With cardiac surgery patients, I had forgotten the simple clinical advice that a rapid decompensation of cardiac function was always cardiac tamponade, unless proven otherwise. In fact, while point-of-care ultrasound is an incredibly powerful diagnostic tool for the modern intensivist, it can also be potentially misleading and dangerous if one simply takes it as truth without overall clinical impression. Clearly, I still had much to learn.

———◆◆———

"Men's hearts failing them for fear" - Luke 21:26

"Red alert," came the call from the crew. "57-year-old lady, ex-smoker. Sudden onset shortness of breath. Saturations on oxygen in the ambulance: 86%. Heart rate 120. Blood pressure 96/40. Temperature 37.4. ETA: 10 minutes."

These were dangerously low saturations. For a woman her age, with no significant past medical history, a sudden onset of shortness of breath with such dramatic vital signs made us think of one key differential diagnosis: pulmonary embolus. A deep vein thrombosis (a blood clot), likely originating in the leg, could have dislodged and made its way to the right side of the heart, then on to the pulmonary circulation. This would cause an obstruction of blood flow to an area of the lung. Without blood flow, no gas exchange occurs, causing low oxygen levels in the blood.

I was doing a stint in A&E at that time. When the pre-alert call came, I prepared myself with the ultrasound machine beside the bed, ready for the patient to arrive. My consultant was also there, curious to confirm the diagnosis himself or support me if I struggled. Two nurses joined us.

Two paramedics, dressed in their dark green uniforms, wheeled Helen into the resuscitation bay from the ambulance. She was gasping for breath, sweaty and panicked. I somehow thought to myself that she somehow didn't look like she had a pulmonary embolus. I wasn't sure why, but I turned to my consultant and caught his eye. He thought the same as I vocalised what I felt. Nevertheless, I wasn't going to merely trust a hunch. Not when I had the ultrasound skills required to confirm it. There was no time for a history. Oxygen. Lots of it. Monitoring attached. Cannula inserted. Ultrasound ready.

"I'm just going to do a quick scan of your heart, Helen," I announced. She nodded, still gasping.

I put the probe onto the middle of her chest. There – on the screen – I saw the heart severely dilated, particularly the left side. It was trying hard to pump, but the muscles had thinned and each pump barely moved the blood into the aorta. Yet, not all of the heart was dilated. The area around the base, near the valves, looked relatively normal.

On another view, the heart looked almost like a balloon, with a narrow base but a large, round apex. I thought to myself that this looked like a specific condition. The Japanese physicians first named it Takotsubo Cardiomyopathy. Takotsubo is the name of the traditional clay jar used to catch octopus. It had a distinctive shape: narrow at its mouth and with a bulbous body. Octopi would swim and crawl into the vessel, which was then lifted from the sea. But while the morphology of the heart was distinctive, the underlying pathology was even more impressive. For Takotsubo cardiomyopathy is also known by several names, including stress cardiomyopathy or broken heart syndrome.

"This is not a pulmonary embolus," I announced after five seconds of putting the probe to the chest, "it's heart failure."

This was the moment, I was sure, the consultant Dom would give me a pat on the back. Surely, he would be impressed by my skill? The speed of diagnosis and certainty with which I differentiated between a pulmonary embolus and heart failure must have been a huge relief for the department that night. In fact, mistaking the conditions for each other may have produced more disastrous consequences.

The emergency treatment for a life-threatening pulmonary embolus would be thrombolysis. This drug "dissolves" blood clots but – as a logical side effect – significantly increases the risk of bleeding. This bleeding may occur in various places, such as the gut or the brain, potentially resulting in catastrophic complications. If we had felt that a pulmonary embolus was likely, we would have given Helen thrombolysis, a treatment which she did not require and could suffer potential complications from. Instead, we started treatment for heart failure, reducing the amount of fluid in the blood vessels and, therefore, the heart, causing it to expend less energy in pumping.

"Yup, could have told you that without the ultrasound," said Dom, before he walked away.

The nurse glanced across the bed at me, then turned away quickly to attach the rest of the monitoring. The silent burn rose from my stomach up into my cheeks. My mouth opened to mutter some sort of smart reply, except my brain failed to conjure anything. Meanwhile, the other registrar saw my embarrassment and, before I could make a fool of myself with some inappropriate comment, announced, "I'm starting the furosemide. Mark, could you grab the CPAP machine, please?"

With my angry thoughts interrupted, I once again focused on the critically ill patient in front of us. Soon, large volumes of urine flowed through the catheter we inserted and out into the collecting bag hung at the side of the trolley; the drug had worked. The tight-fitting mask generated a constant pressure, which not only decreased Helen's breathlessness but also improved heart function. Her blood pressure improved, and her heart rate normalised. Within thirty minutes, her demeanour changed from a panicked frenzy to a calm, collected and comfortable state.

I began to take a history and found out that Helen's husband had left her recently and that she was in large amounts of debt. She had then lost her job due to poor performance. The immense stress of her situation finally broke her heart, literally. This explained the shortness of breath and the heart failure. This was indeed the broken heart syndrome or Takotsubo cardiomyopathy.

When I finally performed a more thorough clinical examination, I indeed saw the signs of heart failure. There were the tall, distended veins on her neck. With my stethoscope to her chest, there were coarse crepitations on the bottom of both her lungs. Likewise, there were the valvular murmurs of a volume-loaded, failing heart.

The signs were there, and my consultant saw them, just as I had done. Perhaps the many more years of experience meant he spotted the diagnosis before I could even see it on the ultrasound, but at that time, I felt that he was jealous of my skills. He, like many other older doctors, did not have the luxury of ultrasound. They had to rely on their clinical examination skills to formulate diagnoses. Well-versed in pattern recognition and clinical acumen built up from decades of experience, they did not require confirmation with a new-fangled technology.

As for a new boy like me, I found my mind trying hard to justify my own skills. I tried to convince myself that the ultrasound was the reason we were confident about one diagnosis over another, that it provided us with confidence to start a treatment plan that could be harmful if we were wrong. I thought about the delay it would have caused if I didn't scan Helen immediately. Perhaps her blood pressure would plummet further. Perhaps she would have had a cardiac arrest. But really, I knew that Dom was right. I would have gotten to the same diagnosis eventually, even without the ultrasound.

While I was caught in my selfish thoughts, the other registrar had already referred Helen to the cardiologists, who admitted her to their coronary care unit. Over the following two weeks, she slowly recovered and eventually went home.

The point-of-care ultrasound enthusiasts (including myself) boast about rapid diagnosis. We come up with many new ways to identify pathology earlier and earlier. We evangelise about the salvation achievable with ultrasound. Yet, many of us know that it is just another tool in our armamentarium. It can sharpen the stethoscope but can equally blunt one's mind into false security. It may identify pathology earlier but may not even confer mortality benefit. It made me feel like a super doctor but did not actually make me a better one.

I continue to teach ultrasound and advocate its use. But after that shift, I took my stethoscope off the door hook in my study. I then walked to the bottom of the garden and placed it against my two hives. We had received another swarm of honeybees in a trap we set up along the side of the house a couple of weeks earlier and had transferred them into another hive adjacent to the first one. With both colonies containing laying queens, there was the collective hum of a queen-rightness; low-pitched, busy and contented. Just as they should be. Perhaps the stethoscope is not dead after all.

"I find your lack of faith disturbing." - Darth Vader, Star Wars

12. Do You Hear the People Sing?

"The lullaby must win" - Jonty Allcock

The depressing sounds of Vanessa's vigil betrayed the signs of spring outside the ICU. The birdsong I heard while cycling into hospital seemed only to tease me into a false sense of security. I could not even sing along to the tunes playing through my earphones. Upon entering the ICU, I was greeted by politely veneered "good mornings" and "hiyas" from the staff. It certainly did not feel like life was about to burst forth. But there seemed to be music constantly emanating from bedspace ten. Tucked away at the corner of the bay, it had been occupied by Vanessa for over a month. A playlist of songs cycled through each day, beckoning me closer as I did my daily review of patients.

Several weeks ago, she was as fit a 35-year-old woman as you could find. She was married with a young child, held a stable job and led an active lifestyle. Then, it began with some muscle aches, then a sniffle, followed by a cough. When the shortness of breath began, she tried her best to cope at home. She put it down to another nursery virus from her little one. Several days went by, and she continued to deteriorate, so the ambulance was called. When she was brought to A&E, it was clear she needed intensive care. Despite intubation and ventilation, though, her oxygen requirements failed to improve. Within a couple of days, the cardiothoracic ICU was called. The ExtraCorporeal Membrane Oxygenation (ECMO) retrieval team made their way to the general ICU to commence ECMO. There was no time to waste; she had already endured almost two weeks of subclinical hypoxia.

Cannulae and pipes, roughly the diameter of one's thumb, were inserted into the femoral vein in the groin for drainage, and in the neck for return of blood. They then formed a circuit with the ECMO pump and oxygenator, which served as a lung machine, allowing oxygen and carbon dioxide to be exchanged across a thin membrane. Curved from the neck and groin towards the ECMO pump sat beside the bed at waist level, the circuit resembled a one-sided silhouette of a violin, except there were no melodies derived from the almost silent revolutions of the pumps. Instead, the regular beeping of her heartbeat on the monitor and the semi-tonal stepwise increase in pitch signified an improvement in blood oxygen saturations and created a strangely reassuring drone of life. This was Vanessa's lifeline, and we protected it at all costs. Unsurprisingly, her lungs soon filled with fluid, a common side effect of ECMO. Her lungs, temporarily relieved of their vital duty, seemed almost to relax into a state of fluidity, making them impossible to ventilate. While the turbine hum from the ventilator continued generating constant pressure, her breaths became smaller until they were only 50ml, the size of a small tumbler.

Number of organ failures: 1

That night, the emergency buzzer sounded. Vanessa. We ran. Peri-arrest. Hurry. The ECMO nurse shouted, "Flow obstruction!"

"Bolus sedation! Grab the Roc[uronium]! 100% oxygen!" I shouted as I fumbled with the plastic gown.

Too late. Cardiac arrest. CPR commenced. Defibrillator pads on. Non-shockable. Adrenaline given. Paralysing agent. Two minutes. Rhythm check. Pulse present!

"Shit. What happened?" I asked.

Vanessa had started to move and coughed. This caused an obstruction to the flow in the ECMO pipes, which then meant her blood oxygen levels plummeted. In turn, her heart struggled with the lack of oxygen and eventually stopped. When it restarted, her blood pressure remained low and required strong infusions to correct it. She was now dependent also on several infusions to maintain her heart function.

Number of organ failures: 2

That was not all. Over the next two days, her kidney function deteriorated rapidly. Acids and toxins accumulated in her body, and yet another machine was wheeled beside bed ten. The green and grey haemofiltration machine stood at the head of the bed next to the ventilator. The vertical collection of infusion pumps towered over the bed at shoulder level. The ECMO machine maintained its position at waist level. Four ominous companions lamenting Vanessa's condition and contemplating her fate as she lay motionless on the bed. There was a constant mumble amongst the vigil. While the drone of the monitor beeped on, the hum of the ventilator turbines, the regular creaks of the infusion pumps and the rubs of the haemofiltration roller pumps on tubing provided a polyphonic, asynchronous and dissonant moan which carried on day and night. This constant nauseating noise of critical illness was occasionally interrupted by various wails from each of the members of the bedside party, only to be rebuked and silenced by the watchful nurse who dutifully changed a syringe or reset an alarm.

Number of organ failures: 3

Days went by, then weeks. Vanessa's husband, Shawn, sick of the constant negative comments of the vigil party, had brought in a music player early on, and it sat on her bedside table. Vanessa had always loved musicals, so this playlist cycled, drowning out the soft mutterings of ongoing life support. While I was sitting in the adjacent bedspace, reviewing another patient, I heard a familiar tune. It was from Victor Hugo's monumental novel turned into one of the most successful musicals, *Les Misérables*.

"Do you hear the people sing, singing the song of angry men. It is the music of a people who will not be slaves again."

I saw *Les Misérables* in the theatre during my first year in medical school. Seated in the last row, I was hardly able to distinguish the two main characters, Javert and Valjean. Unaware of the history of the French Revolution, I had little context with which to place the characters and their stories. I had also only recently arrived in the UK from Singapore and struggled to understand the sung speech and English accents. Little wonder I came out of the theatre completely clueless about the story and felt like I had wasted my money that evening. I didn't revisit *Les Misérables* until several years later when I watched the film version. This time, I was struck by the amazing grace underpinning the story. The undeserving ex-convict Valjean is shown over-the-top grace by a priest when he tries to steal the church's silverware and gets caught red-handed by police officer Javert. This left such a strong impression on Valjean that right at the end of the story, he demonstrated similar grace to Javert despite being discriminated against many times purely based on his criminal history. These concepts were galvanised that same year when I got involved in a small tour with my church's orchestra. We used the same songs to highlight the grace central to the Christian faith. Through these rehearsals and performances, I ended up memorising many of the songs. Now, they seemed to follow me, and as I sat down after my review of another patient, I sang along softly to the music.

Another emergency buzzer. It was Vanessa. I rushed across. She was having a seizure. Several other doctors had arrived. One checked the airway. The other scrutinised the ECMO circuit. Still another did a quick examination, and a fourth administered anti-epileptics. Rapidly, the seizure was controlled, and a CT head scan was booked. When she had stabilised, we brought her down to the scanner, which showed a bleed at the back of her brain.

Number of organ failures: 4

We were stuck. Anticoagulation was needed for ECMO. Without it, blood was likely to clot in the plastic tubing or filters. If this occurred, the ECMO machine could stop working altogether, which would lead very quickly to cardiac arrest. Yet, this same anticoagulation meant that the bleed in Vanessa's brain would likely get worse, and she could die from that instead. In fact, we were concerned that she would not even regain consciousness or cognition. But we had no choice but to stop the anticoagulation.

Shawn was obviously shocked by the news. The machines kept Vanessa alive, but at any time, a clot in the pipes or a further bleed in the brain could spell almost immediate death. We were pessimistic. The cumulative experience of countless deaths and, perhaps more importantly, severely disabled survivors unwittingly tainted our perceptions about recovery potential. With the current technologies in medicine, the term "survival" no longer sufficiently captures the social dilemmas of recovery. What use was it if Vanessa survived but was completely dependent on care? What burden would she impose on family and society in a minimally conscious state? What quality of life might be afforded by the pursuit of survival at all costs?

I saw Shawn walking down the corridor to visit Vanessa one day. The anguish showed in the furrows of his brows. His eyes welled up with each step closer to the bedspace. His head was held high, but his shoulders slouched ever so slightly, hints of the sadness and frustration within. He knelt beside her bed. The four members of the vigil remained towering over them. Both his hands held onto her left hand. His forehead rested down on her hands, and he whispered prayer after prayer as the music played and continued to overwhelm the murmurs of doubt from the vigil and now also from the clinical team.

I felt little hope in my heart. Again, the tune played clearly from the bedside speakers,

"Will you join in our crusade? Who will be strong and stand with me? Beyond the barricade, is there a world you long to see? Then join in the fight that will give you the right to be free."

I did not sing along this time. The massacre which followed the song seemed to be playing out in Vanessa's narrative. I thought of their young child and the mother they were about to lose. Unjust and unfair. This was the limit of medical intervention. She had suffered severe side effects from the machines that kept her alive. Her situation, just like that of the students at the barricade, seemed hopeless. Yet as the music played, each verse seemed like a protest, a build-up for a great victory instead of a terrible defeat. Instead of waving the white flag, Vanessa's banner seemed ever-ready to advance.

"When the beating of your heart matches the beating of the drums, there is a life about to start when tomorrow comes."

Over the next week, Vanessa's body began to recover. Like Valjean emerging from the sewers after saving the half-dead Marius from certain death at the barricade, Vanessa's life was spared, though we had little explanation why. First, her kidneys began to produce urine, and soon, she did not require the help of the kidney machine, which left the room in a grumbling protest of clunky wheels and poor manoeuvrability. One less murmur of doubt.

Number of organ failures: 3

Next, her lungs began to expand over the course of a fortnight. She started to take breaths. Slowly, they became bigger and bigger. First 100mls. A few days later, they were 260mls. By the end of the week, they were 300mls. This was still less than a normal adult breath, but it was sufficient for gas exchange. We tested it by reducing the oxygen supply to the ECMO machine. She coped well. Within a few days, the ECMO machine was no longer needed, and the pipes were removed. One less muttering of fear.

Number of organ failures: 2

Those songs continued to play, willing hope and victory. Each drumbeat seemed to edge her heart back to life. The longer they persisted, the better she became. Gradually, the drugs began to decrease, and the tower was dismantled, one infusion pump at a time. Eventually, the tower was reduced to just a stack of two pumps. Several fewer whispers of despair.

Number of organ failures: 1

A big question remained. Would she wake up with that bleed in the brain? A repeat CT scan still showed the same area of defect, which had clotted by now. It was near the area associated with vision. Would she be blind? Or worse, had she already suffered irreversible brain damage? There was only one way to find out. We weaned the sedation and waited. First, there was a flicker of her fingers. Then, a furrow of her brows. Slowly, her eyes opened after being closed for over a month. I bent over and waved,

"Vanessa, can you hear me? My name is Mark. I'm a doctor here. You are on intensive care."

No response. Just staring. But it was too early to be sure, so I went away and tried again later that day. I thought back to just a week ago. We had tried turning the sedation down, but she had a further seizure. When we tried again after a few days, she failed even to open her eyes but instead bit down on the breathing tube, forcing us to re-sedate her. I didn't hold out much hope for her. Yet, when I went back to her bedspace that afternoon, she looked at me and nodded. I asked her to squeeze my hand. She did, and as I pulled the tube out from her mouth, Vanessa's progress vastly exceeded the entire unit's expectations. She could clearly still see, could hear, could understand and could respond appropriately. We could not explain her recovery. We had no drugs to treat the virus. Somehow, Vanessa's body repaired the damage we thought would be irreversible. Over the next few weeks, she gradually regained her strength. It was the end of spring by now. While some of my other patients had died and several had recovered, few were as dramatic as Vanessa. Springing forth from over a month of dormancy, she had indeed ushered the full bloom of summer. And one day, as I sat in the adjacent bedspace, peering through the window to see her video-calling Shawn, I felt utterly amazed. There, still playing from the speakers at the side of the bed, was her song of victory, her anthem of life, her lullaby of hope,

"Do you hear the people sing, singing the song of angry men? It is the music of a people who will not be slaves again. When the beating of your heart echoes the beating of the drums, there is a life about to start when tomorrow comes." - Les Misérables

[Runner-up for the Society of Medical Writers' Autumn 2022 competition for non-fiction.]

Disability

13. 万箭穿心

万箭穿心 *(wàn jiàn chuān xīn).*
A heart pierced by a thousand arrows.
A Chinese idiom to describe extreme grief.

I remember being taken around the wards by a tutor while preparing for my final medical school exams. During one session, after a short briefing, I was asked to perform a neurological examination of a patient. My heart sank. I feared and hated the neurological exam. There were too many nerves and muscles to remember. Clear instructions were required. Signs were sometimes subtle. Hiding my hesitation, I jumped in and started examining the cranial nerves. I ticked off a mental checklist as I went along:

Cranial nerves I and VII: No change in sense of smell or taste.

Cranial nerves II, III, IV and VI: Pupils equal and reactive, with normal movements.

Cranial nerve V: Sensation seemed normal and so were the muscles of mastication.

Cranial nerve VII: Facial muscles were normal.

Cranial nerve VIII: Hearing seemed grossly normal.

Cranial nerve IX and X: I mentioned I would test the gag reflex.

Cranial nerve XI: Shoulder girdles and neck muscles had good power.

Cranial nerve XII: Tongue movements were normal.

"Hmm," I thought, "nothing to find." This seemed odd since the tutor usually chose patients with physical signs. Undeterred, I thanked the patient and proceeded to present my findings, going through the list of cranial nerves, making sure to use a standard phrase to begin with. This, I was assured by countless others, helped provide an overview and allowed time for the brain to process all the information before needing to synthesise a diagnosis:

"I performed a neurological examination of this patient's cranial nerves. There was no change to her sense of smell or taste. Pupils were equal and reactive. There was no visual field loss or diplopia. The muscles of facial expression were normal.

There was normal sensation and normal muscles of mastication. There was no hearing loss. There were good movements in the neck and shoulders. Tongue movements were normal. In summary, this was a normal cranial nerve examination of this patient."

"That was a pretty good cranial nerves examination," said the tutor, "except you failed to take a step back and notice that there was a set of crutches leaning at the head of the bed. You might have wanted to do a lower limbs examination instead. Do you want to try again?"

My four fellow students could see the shock on my face, followed by a huge sigh of disappointment. Embarrassed, I apologised to the patient for wasting six minutes of her time, asked if I could do another examination, and then proceeded to carefully examine the lower limbs.

Tone: Right leg, normal tone. Left leg, increased tone, feels slightly stiff.

Power: Right leg, normal power. Left leg, mildly weaker in all muscle groups compared to the right.

Sensation: Right leg, normal. Left leg, normal.

Reflexes: Right leg, normal knee and ankle reflexes. Down-going planters. Left leg, subtly increased reflexes, up-going planters.

Coordination: Seemed grossly normal in both legs, allowing for the weakness in power.

Having taken another seven minutes to complete the examination, I began presenting my findings again, followed by a summary and a list of differential diagnoses.

"This patient demonstrates signs consistent with an upper motor neurone lesion. I would like to complete my examination by also examining the upper limbs and cranial nerves, which I have already done. My differential diagnoses include stroke, space-occupying lesion (tumour), or spinal cord pathology."

"That's much better," said the tutor. Addressing the whole group of students, he asked, "Now, suppose we think Miss Smith has had a stroke. Could you tell me what types of stroke you know about and their causes?"

Fortunately, we had prepared for this question recently, so we talked about ischaemic and haemorrhagic strokes. Focusing on ischaemic strokes, we went on to explore the various risk factors and causes. A list was produced eventually. These included:

- Heart disease, including atrial fibrillation, high cholesterol and coronary artery disease
- Hypertension or high blood pressure
- Smoking
- Diabetes
- Obesity
- Increasing age
- Family history
- Being male

Before the 1600s, the understanding of strokes was very poor. It was grouped together with other conditions which cause a disturbance in consciousness, including seizures and head injuries, but also included non-neurological pathologies such as heart attacks or pulmonary embolus (blood clot in the lungs). The umbrella term of "apoplexy" is found in many Hippocratic and Galenic texts, and is associated with non-specific symptoms and signs such as a reduced level of consciousness, groaning, aphasia, or sensory and motor disturbances.

In 1658, Swiss physician Johann Jacob Wepfer wrote a case report about a particular patient on whom he had performed an autopsy. He identified the massive bleeding that caused the patient's *apoplexy* and, by doing so, got to the source of the problem: strokes were a result of vascular problems (either clots or bleeds), not necessarily a problem with the brain tissue itself. The risk factors listed above are indeed mostly associated with vascular problems, from hypertension all the way down to family history.

During my training, I recalled this list one day when I was in the Emergency Department examining a patient. Still, I could not figure out why the woman in front of me exhibited signs of a stroke. She had already experienced a seizure and was now drowsy, but she demonstrated the classic signs of a stroke. There was the clear unilateral facial droop and weakness on one side of her body. There was also dysphasia, an inability to speak coherently or express herself. I was thus unable to get a history from her. There was increased tone and brisk reflexes, just like the patient I examined as a medical student. There was the seizure. All signs of a stroke. However, Lucy was only in her 30s, and she was a slim woman. She didn't have a family history of strokes, nor did she have diabetes or hypertension. She did not smoke. More importantly, she did not even have atrial fibrillation or any previous heart disease. She had none of the textbook risk factors. Why, then, did she have all the signs of a stroke?

I called her name loudly. No response. Then, a firm squeeze of the shoulder to produce pain. Only groans and flickers of her wrists, and her eyes remained closed. A low Glasgow Coma Score (GCS) of seven. I was clearly missing an aetiology, but there wasn't time to think. Lucy started having another seizure. We needed to intubate her. Several colleagues assisted in administering the anaesthesia and intubating Lucy. Once this was done, we swiftly took her to the radiology department for a CT head scan after a quick chest X-ray in the emergency department. Following these, she was brought up to the ICU.

While on the ICU, Lucy's social workers furnished us with further details about her life and wellbeing.

They spoke of her long battle with severe depression and anxiety. They told us about the warden-controlled accommodation where she lived due to her mental health issues. Yet, they also told us that she still held a regular job manning the tills of a supermarket chain. She had few friends and almost no visitors. The social workers knew about her history of self-harm, but she tended to wear long-sleeved tops to cover them up. They told us that she had previously been admitted to hospital several times in the past for such attempts. They added that her depression had been getting worse over the previous two years following the breakdown of a relationship.

Lucy had loved a man. They were in a relationship. Things were beautiful for months. But he, too, had mental health issues himself. When they encountered a rocky period in their relationship, just as any other couple would, he ran away. Did not call her. Did not answer his phone. He was uncontactable, and she was distraught. The frequency of self-harm attempts increased after this. Not only did Lucy cut her wrists and arms with razor blades, but she also stuck sewing needles into her own chest and upper abdominal wall. Her already small world, with the sudden loss of love, imploded. On several occasions, Lucy's social workers would find her unkempt and unclean after being called by the supermarket team when she failed to turn up for work.

Back up on the ICU, we reviewed the CT head scan. This revealed multiple strokes of different ages in various areas on both sides of the brain. This was surprising. A single stroke in a discreet area would explain some of the physical signs she demonstrated, but it seemed that Lucy had been having numerous strokes affecting disparate areas. Both the chest X-ray appearances and the story given by Lucy's social workers prompted us to perform an echocardiogram – an ultrasound examination of the heart. There was the problem. Two needles were seen in it. One needle was lodged in the muscle of the right ventricle. The other needle had been pushed from the surface of the chest, through the entire right side of the heart, into the left side. The tip of the needle sat close to the mitral valve between the two chambers of the left heart. On its end, an oval-shaped blob tethered, flapping to and fro with each heartbeat. The turbulence caused by each heartbeat had thrown off multiple tiny clots (emboli) to distant parts of the body. It also caused further accumulation of clots, further spiralling the already dire pathology.

Digging deeper, we managed to get Lucy's medical records from another hospital. It turned out that this needle in her heart had been there for almost a year. She had presented to them with chest pain after admitting to sticking needles in herself. When they did a CT scan, they found not only the needle in the heart, but several needles lodged within her liver, and many more in the soft and fat tissues. At that time, they had managed to extract three needles from her liver.

A multi-disciplinary team consisting of cardiothoracic (heart and lung) surgeons, cardiology, radiology, mental health, and several allied health professionals met to discuss the case. They were sure that Lucy's risk of further self-harm was high. However, she was able to function normally and did not have many symptoms despite the needle in the heart. They discussed the benefits and risks of removing the needle surgically. It was deemed that the potential risks of open-heart surgery were too high, considering the ongoing risks of further self-harm attempts and the lack of symptoms then. The team thus decided that surveillance was the best option for the ongoing management of Lucy. Therefore, she was booked in for several clinic appointments and echocardiograms. She was followed up at three, six and nine months after this episode, and at each appointment, her echocardiogram showed no changes. She was still self-harming occasionally but less frequently than before. There were no new needles in the heart. She held a stable job and seemed to be getting along with life... until this episode.

Many ancient civilisations described a heart-centred physiology. That is, the heart, they believed, was the centre of the body – the most important organ – the sun of the cosmos (in ancient Greek philosophy), and the monarch of the city (in traditional Chinese philosophy).

Ancient Egyptian hieroglyphics portrayed the heart as a jar with several exit tubings. These tubings then carry blood to the rest of the body. Viewed as the most important organ, it was logical for the ancients to ascribe human emotions to the heart. After all, the physical manifestation of intense emotions tends to be an ache in the chest.

Ancient physicians such as Galen, along with the entire Stoical movement, believed that emotions originated from the heart.[24] These thoughts were transmitted to Classical Roman beliefs.[25] Similarly, traditional Ayurvedic medicine believes in the heart as the source of emotions.[26] Likewise, a Chinese term for sadness consists of characters which describe an "injured heart"; 伤心 (shāng xīn), while happiness is directly translated as an "open heart"; 开心 (kāi xīn). Like the Chinese term 心疼 (xīn téng), Lucy's heart swelled with emotion and longing for a loved one. "疼" is used as a verb to dote on a loved one as well as a noun to describe a physical ache. Not dissimilar to the English equivalent

[24] Singer P. Galen Stanford: Stanford University; 2016 [Dec 2019]. Available from: https://plato.stanford.edu/entries/galen/#Mind.

[25] Isidore. The Etymologies of Isidore of Seville. Cambridge: Cambridge Unviersity Press; c.615-630.

[26] Porter R. The greatest benefit to mankind: a medical history of humanity from antiquity to the present. London: HarperCollins; 1997.

of "heartache", the term describes the seemingly physical ache in one's chest as a response to intense emotional distress.

Classical Latin words such as "cardiaca" demonstrate the explicit link between heart disease and emotional turmoil. Isidore's famous work *Etymologies* describes it as a "suffering of the heart accompanied by terrible fear". Believing in a heart-centred physiology, Isidore describes the heart as a governing or pivotal force of human action by drawing similarities between the heart (cardia) and a door hinge (cardo).

In the Hindu Charaka Samhita (2nd century CE), the heart upholds the physical integrity of the body. It is likened to the foundation beam of a house, much like the building concept of a cornerstone. As the seat of consciousness, the heart not only governs emotions but provides an intrinsic link to cognition. It goes further by suggesting the avoidance of mental stress to protect cardiac health. The interplay between emotions and cognition is similarly well demonstrated in the ancient Greek myth of Cupid as the god of erotic love and desire. Along the development of history, the bow and arrow and a torch became Cupid's iconic weapons. His victims' hearts would be pierced and inflamed, finally resulting in surrender to their uncontrollable desires. Stirred through strong emotions, the victims would thus "fall" in love, exhibiting reckless abandon, foolish action and unbreakable resolve. Perhaps it was this emotion which caused Lucy to stick needles into herself.

Lucy's CT head scan demonstrated many areas of brain damage. It was obvious that the source was the small blood clot which had formed at the tip of the needle in her heart. Unsurprisingly, Lucy failed to wake up in the days following the stroke. Her brain had suffered irreversible damage to multiple areas. Each time we tried to turn down the sedative agents keeping her asleep, she would make some un-purposeful movements, take inadequate breaths and slowly start to desaturate due to lack of oxygen in her blood going to her tissues.

Lucy's higher respiratory centres had been damaged. These areas control the automaticity of breathing, varying the rate and volume of breaths according to markers in the blood. We had to control her breathing to allow sufficient oxygen to be delivered to her tissues and organs. Several attempts were made to wean the sedation and ventilator support. It was time to change our priorities. Clearly, Lucy's actions were slaves to her emotions. Master of her life, she felt each setback in the middle of her chest, each disappointment reaffirming and resonating with the last. Like countless others in history, Lucy felt each emotional pang deep in her heart.

Much like Cupid's arrow, Lucy's heart was literally inflamed by the needle which pierced it. Not merely an emotional override of normal inhibitions, as in the case of Cupid's victims, Lucy's condition was far more pathological. Her uninhibited actions of self-harm caused further loss of control of not only her conscious actions, but all her basic physiological functions. Lucy was unable to speak, move, or even breathe on her own.

A personification of the Chinese idiom, Lucy's heart was pierced by "arrows", manifestations of the grief she faced daily.

The damage had been done.

Her fate was sealed.

A heart pierced by "arrows" – lost to love – finally gave up on the grief and the struggle of life itself.

> *Why does my heart go on beating?*
> *Why do these eyes of mine cry?*
> *Don't they know it's the end of the world?*
> *It ended when you said goodbye*
> *- The End of the World by Skeeter Davis*

14. Spice

"The spice must flow..." Frank Herbert's Dune

Prison was like Arrakis for the young, 20-year-old Luke. The concrete, windowless cells much like the barren landscape of the fictional desert planet in Frank Herbert's 1965 science fiction epic, *Dune*. Exiled to Her Majesty's Pleasure for a minor offence, Luke did not quite grasp the trouble that awaited. In fact, he was impressed by how "friendly" the other prisoners were. Within a few days of being there, they started offering him cigarettes. But these were not regular tobacco.

They called it "bird-killer". "Bird" as in "birdlime", historically a sticky gum spread on branches to trap small birds. Like for trapped birds, they said it helped them kill time serving their long sentences. On the street, though, this same drug is much better known as "spice". Spice, the same drug which lies at the heart of the *Dune* story. Unlike in *Dune*, however, Luke's encounter with spice did not afford him prescience nor the ability to navigate time and space.

It wasn't Luke's first time trying cannabis, but he was completely unaware of the potency of its synthetic cousin. Within an hour of smoking spice, he felt relaxed, sinking deeper and deeper into a hole of apathy, a distinct numbing of his senses which helped him forget his predicament. The other prisoners didn't seem quite as sedate as he was becoming. But that was the extent of his memory. Soon, he was unrousable and barely breathing. Slumped by his bed, the prison guards knew exactly what he had taken. The doctor was called, and soon, this was escalated, and Luke was brought to A&E.

By the time he arrived in A&E, it had already been hours since Luke smoked that joint. The paramedics had tried to support his breathing. They gave him naloxone, a reversal agent for opioid toxicity, not knowing what he had taken. But this only had a transient effect. They gave him oxygen to maximise delivery to his tissues. They gave him fluids to boost his low blood pressure. The A&E staff realised that these were insufficient and prepared to intubate him. Only small boluses of drugs were needed to render Luke anaesthetised, after which the team successfully intubated, ventilated and inserted lines to maintain sedation. A quick detour through the CT scanner was made before Luke landed in ICU.

In ICU, after initial stabilisation and the setting up of all the machines, the nurses and healthcare assistants washed, changed, shaved, brushed and cleaned the prisoner, all while two police officers continued to keep watch over his ICU prison cell. The smell of spice was fortunately soon replaced by Old Spice,[27] thanks to the ironic sense of humour of staff nurse Steven.

Luke's CT scan did not show any obvious pathology in his brain. However, CT scans cannot pick up cellular damage caused by tissue hypoxia. This was quite clearly the case when – days down the line – we were trying to wake Luke up, and all he did was violently flail his limbs without purpose. Each time we tried to wean the sedative drugs, he would flail, but without purposeful movements. His breathing pattern became erratic, his blood pressure shot up, and his limbs threatened to break all the lines attached to him. On a couple of instances, the police officers had to help control his movements while we reintroduced sedation. Different agents were tried in various combinations. Finally, with a high dose of an alternative sedative, dexmedetomidine, he settled.

Through speaking to the police officers, I soon found out that smuggling of spice into the prison was rampant. Many of the prisoners were addicted, but due to the various methods of disguising it, it was almost impossible for the prison guards to prevent its use. At first, due to its legal status, spice would be sprayed onto actual dried rolled cannabis leaves and sent in envelopes to the prisoners. They reminded me of the rolled Chinese tea leaves of my ancestors: 铁观音 (tie guan yin).[28] Named after the Buddhist goddess of mercy, 观音 (guan yin), this was perhaps fitting imagery for the unconditional love and relief of suffering that this deity bestowed upon even the lowest criminals.

---

[27] Old Spice is an American brand of men's deodorant, famous for their humorous and sometimes provocative TV advertisements.

[28] 铁观音 (tie guan yin) tea originates from Fujian province. This was where my forefathers lived before my great grandparents emigrated to Singapore.

Ironically, these days, many street drugs in the UK, including spice, originate from China.[29] A side effect of globalisation is the ease with which people can obtain chemicals and drugs. Online black markets buzz with activity. Vendors sell their goods based on chemical structure. UK buyers (such as drug dealers) get sent packages of powder to press into pills or dissolve into solutions. Without specialist labs such as those in universities and forensic departments, there is almost no way to verify the purity or exact chemicals within these packages. Furthermore, legislation cannot keep up with the various novel chemicals produced. When one compound does become illegal, it stimulates a flurry of activity to create alternative substances. As a result, further substances are created, with sometimes undesirable effects or extreme potency. Little wonder why the "legal high" market is impossible to control.

As the legislation around spice tightened, the smuggled forms became more and more creative. Soon, the prisoners' friends realised that spice would dissolve in the acetone of nail polish remover. The dissolved spice would then be sprayed onto personal letters and sent to the prisoners. These would initially bypass the normal security and search measures. The prisoners would then cut small squares of the paper, mix them in with tobacco roll-up cigarettes and smoke them, achieving the desired effect. Soon, the prison guards caught on to the trick, and they would search and test all personal letters for the drug. To continue their habit, fake legal letters were sent to the prisoners, impregnated with spice like before. Because they were "legal letters", the prison guards were not allowed to open them, and thus, the prisoners continued to receive their drugs.

To determine the dosage of the spice-laden letters, seasoned prisoners would use the newbies as guinea pigs, offering them the narcotic and observing the effect before partaking themselves. However, the spraying and hanging process would result in higher concentrations of cannabinoids towards the bottom of the letter, and lower concentrations toward the top. Likewise, the heavier impregnated leaves would make their way

---

[29] MacKenzie C, Novel Psychoactive Substances. ANWICU Lakes Meeting; 2019; Windemere: Association of North West ICUs.

to the bottom of the packet of leaves, resulting in a magnitude of physical manifestations dependent on which part of the product was used. Unfortunately, Luke must have received the wrong end of the letter and used spice up to 80 times the potency of natural cannabinoids. The stupor which resulted starved not only his perception but also the oxygen supply to his brain. Three days after admission into ICU, a repeat CT scan and EEG were performed for persistent poor neurological function. Both demonstrated features of hypoxic brain injury. There was little hope of recovery for this young man.

The following day, we extubated Luke. While he was able to breathe for himself, he was only minimally conscious. Simply unable to obey commands, it left us with little confidence about his recovery potential. A couple of days went by, and Luke continued to be agitated, uncontrollably moving his limbs in regular myoclonic jerks. He was moved to a floor mattress for fear of an inadvertent fall out of bed. He required a staff member to always be present to prevent self-injury.

Regular sedatives soon controlled his flailing but reduced him to an empty shell. His limbs would make few movements. His jaw regularly opened and closed in circular movements, causing his teeth to grind constantly. Loud, long moans were heard frequently, and while his eyes roamed around without ever fixing, tears would occasionally be seen trickling down his cheek. Unable to eat or drink, nutrition was provided through the nasogastric tube, bridled, like the nose ring of a cow, to prevent dislodgement.

After a few more days, the nasogastric tube was replaced by a percutaneous gastrostomy tube, which permitted access directly to the stomach via a tube which communicated with the surface of the skin of the abdomen. The urinary catheter was replaced with adult diapers.

Within a week, Luke was stepped down to the ward, a mere shadow of the man he once was. He had swapped Her Majesty's Prison for a mental solitary confinement, where his minor sentence had become one for life. The squalor of his cell was replaced by the darkness of a brain damaged beyond cognition or control, trapped in an unfortunate Nirvana. Extinguished, spent and shelled, young Luke was eventually discharged to a nursing home, where the severity of his condition made even the geriatric residents comparatively thankful for their own predicament.

I looked at Luke upon his discharge. A "success" of medicine: mortality 0, survival 1. Yet, I could not help but despair. In his curiosity, Luke fell victim to the manipulation of his seasoned inmates. I thought of John William Waterhouse's painting *Sleep and his half-brother Death*, which hinted at the fine line between recreational opioid use and toxicity. In reference to the Greek gods Hypnos (sleep) and Thanatos (death), *Sleep* is personified as a young man, lounging and sleeping semi-reclined on a comfortable couch. He is tranquil, clutching a poppy in this hand as an acknowledgement of the somniferous effects of the opiates contained in the seedpod. His legs are crossed, and his top draped lazily across his chest, exposing one of his nipples. There is a sense of rest and relaxation in the character of *Sleep*. Beside him, within the darkness, lies his half-brother, *Death*. *Death* is portrayed in a similarly restful state. His eyes are closed, his head tilted backwards, and his arm nestled under *Sleep*. *Death* could easily have been mistaken for *Sleep* in the painting if not for the darkness that surrounds him. In the foreground, opium pipes hint at the underlying message of the painting. Much like Luke, there is a very fine, sometimes blurred line between *Sleep* and *Death* afforded by narcotics. Another quote from American poet Bayard Taylor captured the far-reaching sequelae of opioid misuse,

"And far and wide, in a scarlet tide, the poppy's bonfire spread."

The effects of drug-induced sedation did not seem quite as still or serene as what Waterhouse portrayed. Instead, Luke was stuck in a state beyond both sleep and death. The wails, weeping and gnashing of teeth seemed an unjust eternal punishment for a young man dragged down by the scum of the earth. Back in prison, the spice continued to flow, the memory of Luke was consumed by the sand, another victim of the worm that does not die, and the fire that is not quenched.

"A poison so subtle, so insidious, so irreversible…"
- Frank Herbert's Dune

15. Flaccidity

"It is, as far as he knows, the only way to go downstairs…"
Winnie the Pooh, by A.A. Milne

There is a helplessness about flaccidity. A slumped, sighing, throwing-in-the-towel resignation about the loss of muscular tone. The deep, dark embarrassment it exudes from its association with sexual impotence. The tail-between-your-legs feeling of not living up to expectations or standards. But these are just the head of the problem. Further down the shaft… I mean body, flaccidity can also act as a harbinger of far more sinister pathology. This is the case in the initial stages of a stroke, when a part or entire side of the body goes limp – external manifestations of a significant clot or bleed within the brain.

Yet whole body flaccidity strangely seems to provoke humorous depictions instead of dread, sometimes. I remember reading Winnie the Pooh to my 3-year-old daughter. She would laugh uncontrollably at the "bump, bump, bump" description of Pooh's flaccid descent down the stairs, useless and limp at the mercy of Christopher Robin. Upon hearing her laughter, I could not help but laugh myself. Yet, after reading Viktor Frankl's terrible description of dead bodies being dragged by fellow exhausted prisoners in a similar fashion from the typhoid tent up the stairs to the mortuary, I could not bear to read that passage in Winnie the Pooh in the same way anymore. The "bump, bump, bump" of real human heads upon concrete steps became all too haunting to me.

I visualised the grim, gaunt and gloomy prisoners, severely malnourished, with insufficient energy to even carry their fellow prisoners up a few steps. I remembered the strange, queasy feeling I experienced walking through Auschwitz, the weight of countless deaths stirring through my very bowels. I imagined the blood that had been smeared over those concrete steps to the mortuary. Those few inanimate steps gloated victory over the flaccidity and impotence of the swathes of previously healthy men, women and children who succumbed to torture, malnutrition and disease. Far closer to home, I am also reminded of the terrible flaccid conditions we see in the ICU.

Flaccidity was the initial catalyst for the development of intensive care medicine. Poliomyelitis is a virus affecting the motor nerves. Flaccid, atrophic limbs are characteristic of milder infections, and have been depicted even in ancient Egyptian frescos. Severe infections of the central nervous system can sometimes result in complete paralysis, whether temporary or permanent. This stimulated the invention of the iron lung in the late 1920s, a huge machine which engulfs the entire patient's body (except the head) and generates a rhythmic vacuum, helping them to breathe. No longer did medical students or nurses need to ventilate such patients by hand. Instead, a machine provided a surrogate for the normal respiratory cycle. When a vacuum was generated inside the cavity, the patient's chest would expand. This was a breath. When the vacuum was released, the chest fell as the patient exhaled. Some polio patients recovered after a few weeks and were able to breathe for themselves. During this time, the iron lung literally maintained their lives. Unfortunately, some patients never recovered and spent the rest of their lives within the iron lung.

In 1952, a particularly bad polio epidemic hit Europe, resulting in many hundreds of patients becoming severely paralysed.[30] Again, medical students were called to assist in ventilating patients by hand. The prohibitive costs and sheer bulk of the iron lung meant there were insufficient units to cope with the demand. This need, along with the unsustainable use of medical students as ventilators, resulted in the adoption of positive pressure ventilators (which were already used in anaesthesia then) for such patients. These machines are far more compact and mechanically simpler than iron lungs. Instead of creating a vacuum to stimulate breathing, they blew air into the lungs. They could thus be connected to the patient via tubing instead of enveloping the entire patient – a far more elegant alternative to the iron lung. This epidemic then stimulated the need for such patients to be managed in a specialised unit – the beginnings of the intensive care unit. It is no wonder that the perception of intensive care is one steeped in complex machinery. Yet, despite the multidisciplinary aspects of critical care and the multitude of

---

[30] BBC. History of Polio London: British Broadcasting Corporation; 2015 [Available from: https://www.bbc.co.uk/news/health-17045202.

machines contained within our armamentarium, the ventilator continues to maintain its central position within the public's view of intensive care medicine.

———•••———

Thanks to vaccinations against polio, I have never needed to care for a patient with this dreadful disease. But there are some similarly disruptive pathological syndromes we see on a regular basis in the ICU.

Robert first experienced the typical muscle aches and fatigue of a viral infection in early winter. He thought little of it, putting it down to a minor cold virus. Even after several days, the diarrhoea felt more like an inconvenience rather than a worry. In fact, he did recover after about a week and continued pottering around his garden with his little white dog, preparing his plants for winter.

Robert was a retired engineer. At 78 years of age, he continued to maintain his active lifestyle. He would play tennis weekly with some friends. He did his own shopping. He even mowed his own lawn in the summer. To him, the virus was hardly a setback. But two weeks after he first developed symptoms, he continued to feel weak and fatigued. In fact, despite the muscle aches and diarrhoea resolving, he felt weaker than ever before.

First, he noticed that going upstairs to bed was exhausting. Then, making a cup of tea was difficult. Finally, he became short of breath even while watching television. He called 999. When the paramedics arrived, they noticed he was unable to speak in full sentences. The coarse crackles of fluid within his lungs were barely heard, only on account of his poor inhalation effort. Something was not right. By the time the oxygen saturations probe displayed a reading of 88% on the monitor, they already knew he was critically ill.

Oxygen was rapidly administered. Robert was put onto a trolley and brought into the ambulance. The blue lights were turned on. Off they sped to the hospital. En route, the red phone rang in A&E. This was reserved for pre-alert patients; ones the paramedics are concerned about.

"78-year-old gentleman. Shortness of breath. Heart rate 108. BP (blood pressure) 146/96. Saturations 88% on air, 95% on non-rebreathe mask.[31] GCS 14.[32] ETA: Ten minutes," reported the paramedic over the phone.

The A&E team assessed Robert and immediately recognised that he was in respiratory distress. His blood gas sample results supported this. His respiratory effort was poor, and he was hardly able to cough. His blood oxygen levels were so low that if we had left him, he would rapidly deteriorate and die. Furthermore, his carbon dioxide levels were very high. Normally, breathing faster and harder would rid the body of carbon dioxide, but Robert was unable to do so.

I was summoned as the ICU registrar on call.

As with many of our patients, it was clearly impossible to get a history from Robert. Not only was he confused from the lack of oxygen, he was also unable to speak more than a single word with each breath. With each forceful attempt at inhalation, his chest struggled to expand sufficiently. As with many of our patients who suffer from pneumonia, they get to a point where they are too tired to carry on breathing sufficiently. Exhausted, their blood oxygen levels fall, and carbon dioxide rises. Without intervention, the carbon dioxide levels eventually reach the point of loss of consciousness. After this, death ensues.

We quickly prepared for intubation and mechanical ventilation. Without a history, we had assumed Robert suffered from a severe pneumonia. He had the runny nose and the initial fatigue of an infection, followed by gradual deterioration over days to weeks. Indeed, his chest X-ray showed areas of dense infection: a term called consolidation. Instead of the fluffy air-filled space of the tiny air sacs of the lungs, Robert's were filled with inflammatory and infective slush. This was simply unconducive for gas exchange.

There was no time to waste, and we very quickly got the kit and the personnel to intubate Robert. As always, a checklist was

---

[31] This mask is connected to a reservoir bag. It allows the bag to be filled with oxygen. The patient then breathes in from this reservoir, enabling a high concentration of oxygen to be delivered. Usually, 15 litres per minute of oxygen is pumped into the bag.

[32] The Glasgow Coma Scale (GCS) is a widely used scoring system of level of consciousness. Scores are given for eye, verbal and motor responses. A normal score is 15. 14 represented the state Robert was in, one point deducted for his confused verbal responses.

used to ensure we did not forget anything in such an emergency. From the doctor performing the intubation to the runner, all check. From the drugs used for induction of anaesthesia to those needed to maintain it, check. From the best-case scenario of successful intubation to the worst-case scenario of an emergency tracheotomy, check.

It didn't take much to get Robert off to sleep. He had been clearly obtund since we arrived in A&E. Soon, he was intubated, put on the ventilator and started on potent antibiotics. His blood gas parameters soon improved dramatically. So dramatically that the next day, he was needing minimal amounts of oxygen and was taking good breaths with minimal help from the ventilator. We extubated him.

Another life saved. Or so we thought.

Within hours, Robert began to look increasingly sweaty. He struggled to breathe and soon looked exhausted. His blood gas parameters returned to a similar state as the one taken in A&E. We re-intubated him. After a further two days, we again weaned him off the ventilator and extubated him. Yet again, he was unable to maintain sufficient respiratory effort. He looked clammy and distressed. His eyes were wide with fear of suffocation. And he was, since his oxygen levels on the blood gas were dangerously low, and his carbon dioxide very high. His respiratory pattern was awful, and he began to cough frothy sputum, suggesting an element of pulmonary oedema.[33]

We needed to re-intubate him, fast.

I managed the airway, while my consultant administered the drugs, and another junior doctor kept her eyes fixed on the monitor, titrating the noradrenaline infusion to counter the wild swings in blood pressure. Again, once on the ventilator, Robert's parameters improved rapidly and dramatically. But we dared not attempt a further extubation, so we performed a tracheostomy two days later. Then, when all the sedation was weaned the

---

[33] Pulmonary oedema describes fluid within the alveoli of the lungs. A common cause of this is left heart failure, but it can also happen with airway obstruction. The lungs generate negative pressure to draw more air, but due to the obstruction, instead of air being drawn in, fluid is drawn out of the capillaries, into the alveoli. The feeling of suffocation from either cause is severely distressing for patients.

following day, we noticed that his limbs were unable to move. All four limbs were completely paralysed.

We got very worried.

I was initially concerned that during my re-intubation, the neck extension may have caused a cervical spinal cord injury. After all, he was elderly and may have already had degenerative spinal disease that we had not known about. The fragile, irregular, osteoarthritic vertebra may have impinged on the spinal cord during intubation, causing permanent injury. More unlikely was critical illness-related weakness. It was far too early in his stay for this, far too soon for his muscles to atrophy. Robert had no previous record of neurological conditions, so this was not a flare-up of an underlying condition. Or perhaps it was a stroke. We scanned his head. The scan was negative.

On return from the scan, Robert then began to develop wildly labile blood pressures. Within seconds, for no discernible reason, they would plummet to levels so low that the nurses immediately pulled the emergency buzzer. But before the defibrillator arrived for the impending cardiac arrest, they would recover spontaneously. Meanwhile, the noradrenaline infusion, which we had increased to raise his blood pressure, would then cause severe hypertension, threatening to result in the rupture of blood vessels in the brain. Then, as quickly as it began, the blood pressure would settle by itself.

We then remembered one nugget of information handed over by the paramedics: he had a viral infection a week prior to his admission. It finally dawned on us that Robert was suffering from a neurological condition called Guillain-Barre Syndrome. It wasn't the infection that had caused these severe symptoms, nor my heavy-handed emergency intubation attempt, but his own body.

Also known as an autoimmune post-infective neuropathy, Guillain-Barre Syndrome results from the body producing antibodies against its own nerves. Robert's immune system, activated by the microscopic particles of the virus, produced a targeted reaction against it. However, the antibodies produced against this virus unfortunately bore close resemblance to his nerve tissues. As a result, his immune system began to attack his own nerves.

This explained the initial weakness. It also explained the respiratory distress. Slowly, his nerves were unable to function properly, causing progressive weakness, which began in his legs and ascended all the way up to his chest, finally paralysing even his respiratory muscles. In addition, the nerves which normally controlled the muscular tone of Robert's blood vessels and the rhythm of his heart were affected. This was the reason for the large swings in blood pressure and heart rate. A lumbar puncture was performed. The clear-looking cerebrospinal fluid, in fact, contained high concentrations of protein, confirming the diagnosis.

Flaccid from the neck down, Robert was completely dependent on the ventilator for his breathing. For weeks, he remained almost completely paralysed. Day by day, he became more and more depressed. The daily assessment of muscular strength was a reminder of how powerless he was. The regular neurological tests highlighted his utter impotence and incompetence. The many doctors, nurses, physiotherapists, and dietitians on ward rounds became audiences for his abysmal, motionless performance. Instead of rapturous applause received by John Cage, Robert's daily 4'33"[34] performance was invariably met with shakes of heads and deep frowns. He could not even twitch his fingers or toes. Gradually, his muscles themselves began to atrophy from disuse, and he began to get pressure sores from his inability to shift in the bed. His bony prominences tented the slack skin, which seemed ever ready to fall to the ground. If not for the movements in his face and the attempts at breathing aided by the ventilator, Robert could as well be rotting. This surely was flaccidity at its most feeble.

One day, during my daily review of Robert, he stared at me and started mouthing words. His tracheostomy meant he was unable to produce any sounds, but with his lips, he tried to communicate. I struggled to lip-read. I guessed each word. Most

---

[34] John Cage composed his notoriously controversial piece 4'33" in 1952. For the duration of 4 minutes and 33 seconds, performers would stay silent and sometimes motionless at their instruments. The BBC4 performance of this piece in 2013 saw an entire orchestra in silence for the stipulated duration, followed by thunderous applause from a sell-out crowd.

were wrong. I asked if he was in pain. He wasn't. Unable to even write, he had little option but to repeat himself.

As I leaned in closer, I noticed several features that made me lament his current fate and wonder about his future prognosis. His facial muscles had lost their bulk. His eyes, sunken in their sockets, no longer held the depths of his soul. Instead, I felt as though I looked straight through his skull. The normal pink tinge of health was absent from his cheeks. In its place was a pale shade of grey skin which lacked the warmth of life. The patchy, uneven stubble on his chin made Robert look haggard, unkempt, and uncared for. His lips, dry, cracked and pale, seemed a fitting manifestation of the mental and emotional wilderness he was stuck in. Likewise, his breath stank of resignation, of surrender, and of despair. This was a man who had already given up.

"L..." he mouthed.

"Let?" I asked. A nod.

"M..."

"Me?" another nod.

"D...Die..."

He knew I had finally got it. In his eyes, a kindling of flame appeared for a second, hope that we would be able to end his suffering immediately. I did not share his hope. His hope was for euthanasia. My hope was for his recovery. Yet, I felt deeply saddened by his predicament. Within a couple of weeks, an able-bodied man was reduced to a near skeleton. Robert was essentially useless in his flaccid and impotent state. He could not enjoy life, nor could he contribute to society. He was unable to control his basic functions of eating, drinking or excreting. He was just as helpless as the polio victims, dependent on their iron lung. Just as hopeless as the prisoners in Auschwitz.

"You know I can't, Robert. We've talked about this before," I said while shaking my head. "Besides, there has been some progress. You're needing less help from the ventilator compared to a few weeks earlier. You were able to move your little finger this morning, remember? We know that the majority of patients with this condition recover, and I know it feels like forever, but there is still hope."

I stayed with him for a further few minutes, highlighting the progress he had already made. I reminded him about his garden and his dog, at least two things to look forward to after recovery. I sat at the edge of the bed and held his hand. I told him about my own faith and beliefs. He began to cry. I stayed a few minutes longer.

Over the next couple of weeks, we tried our best to improve his mood. We encouraged him with even the millimetres of movement he regained in his fingers. We reminded him that his lungs were working well and that he needed less help from the ventilator. The nurses washed and combed his hair and shaved his face a couple of times a week. On a quiet day on the unit, we even managed to take him outside of the hospital for a change of scenery. This was no mean feat. Because Robert was dependent on the ventilator, we had to ensure adequate oxygen and power supply for it. He continued to have labile blood pressures, so required several infusion pumps to be always connected. The monitoring had to be taken with us. In the end, all the spare equipment and supplies had to be piled onto a separate metal procedural trolley. Three nurses came along. One ensured all the connections and monitors were secure as we moved, while another helped to open doors. The third nurse pushed the ventilator while I pushed the bed. It took over an hour to get to the garden of the hospital from the time we started preparing.

The grey, overcast skies surely did not inspire much joy for me. However, the mere change of scenery from the angular, claustrophobic, and sterile environment of the ICU to the green, irregular, and organic features of the hospital garden seemed to stir a renewed spirit within Robert. For several days after that somewhat cumbersome excursion, Robert cooperated far more readily with the physiotherapists and pushed himself with various exercises. His ventilator settings improved. He felt less pain. There was a pinkness in his face that was missing a week prior.

The following week, we managed to bring Robert's dog into the ICU to visit him. Another junior doctor, Nadine, wrote to several teams and managed to gain approval for this form of animal-assisted therapy. Robert was overjoyed to see his small, white, fluffy Maltese dog. In fact, the rest of the staff were just as excited to have an animal in the ICU, and so were the other conscious patients. Again, for several days, the joy of seeing his dog lingered, reflected by Robert's compliance with physiotherapy and further improvements in his neurological status.

It had been two months since Robert was admitted to the ICU. Slowly, he had regained strength in his arms, but still had little to no movement in his legs. His respiratory muscles had recovered, and he was able to breathe through the tracheostomy with some supplemental oxygen but without needing the support of the ventilator. He had overcome the recurrent chest infections from spending time on the ventilator, the pressure sores on his sacrum and the constant burning sensation of neuropathic pain in his feet. He was finally ready for us to remove his tracheostomy. While this was done with little fanfare for us, I was sure it felt like a hard-won victory for Robert. There was tangible hope. No longer was he connected to a machine for breath. No longer was he mute. No longer did he need ICU. The small "step-down"[35] to the ward was, in fact, a giant leap for Robert.

Robert spent a further few months in hospital before gaining sufficient strength to go home for further rehabilitation. He was just about able to walk with a frame upon his departure from the hospital.

■ ◆ ◆ ■

One cannot examine such helpless paralysis without paying homage to the ex-editor of Elle magazine, Jean-Dominique Bauby. Poignant were his observations about the struggles of paralytic conditions in his incredible book about his experiences with locked-in syndrome, entitled *The Diving Bell and the Butterfly*.

Bauby suffered from a brainstem stroke, which left him completely paralysed, aside from the ability to blink. Despite this, his brain function was normal. He was completely conscious and oriented but could not demonstrate any movement or overt signs. His doctors initially thought he was in a vegetative or minimally conscious state, but through further investigations, they realised that he was indeed fully awake and neurologically

---

[35] We use the term "step-down" to refer to a patient going to the ward from ICU. Since the care within hospitals is graded in ascending numbers with the increasing needs of the patient, ICU is often considered a "higher level" of care, or an "escalation" of care.

intact. Stuck in the empty shell of a body, Bauby eventually learnt to live with his condition and wrote a book with the help of his assistant. The assistant would repeatedly recite the frequency-ordered alphabet and Bauby would blink when she got to the letter he wanted next. The entire process took two months, working up to three hours a day and seven days a week.

I re-read the book following my encounter with Robert and felt completely moved by the mental explorations of this otherwise helpless character. Despite Bauby's physical cocoon, his mind travelled far and wide. Despite being fed exclusively via a feeding gastrostomy, he continued to partake in viscerally exquisite fine dining experiences. Despite the inability to speak, his words penetrated far deeper into the hearts of many, perhaps more so than when he was editor of Elle.

I just wished I had thought about reading a copy of the book to Robert during his stay with us or, better still, getting the DVD for the TV, which was always on by the side of his bed. Perhaps then he would not merely be confined to the "bump, bump, bump" of total flaccidity. Instead, during the many weeks in ICU, and then months in rehabilitation, Robert might have been enjoying "hunny", getting stuck in rabbit holes from gluttony, playing imaginary Pooh-sticks, humming silly tunes, and exploring the Hundred Acre Wood.

16. The Worst Scars are in The Mind

"The worst scars are in the mind" - Hernán Reyes,
International Charter of the Red Cross

"[Torture], like pornography, is easier to recognise than it is to define."
Paraphrased from Griselda Cooper, Fundamental Principles and
Practice of Anaesthesia

Imagine days or weeks of isolation, no semblance of day or night, without family, friends or loved ones. Imagine not eating or drinking, unable to speak or clean, stripped naked and forced into various postures. Imagine being sedated, tranquillised, and semi-conscious in a seemingly never-ending process of dying.

The International Charter of the Red Cross' review on psychological torture makes for a haunting read. Halfway through the review, the author invites the reader into a disturbingly detailed exploration of several documented psychological torture methods. It sends shivers down my spine. I need not reproduce the methods here, for they are remarkably similar to many of the environmental conditions and interventions in the intensive care unit.

Isolated from their families, many patients spend days or weeks on ICU, dependent on a ventilator. Sedated, in suspenseful unrest instead of comfortable slumber. Frequently disturbed by observations and interventions. Disrupted day-night cycles. Occasionally paralysed. Unable to eat or drink, nutrition is often delivered directly into the stomach via a feeding tube, a poor substitute for the sustenance and sensory stimulation of a proper meal. Little wonder why many patients wake up confused and disoriented: a state we call delirium.

The manifestations of delirium are diverse, from the exuberant to the subdued, from the physically violent to the verbally abusive, from the paranoid to the sexually inappropriate. Despite the recognition of the syndrome as early as the 1st century CE by Celsus, we still know disappointingly little about delirium. We have identified predisposing factors, and we know to avoid certain drugs, but many of the studies into its prevention have failed to demonstrate significant progress. This is partly due to the multitude of factors that contribute to delirium.

The darkness of delirium seems – for many victims – coloured by their personalities, providing voyeuristic glimpses into their deepest fears or inhibitions. This was especially the case with Bob, who had bowel perforation where faecal contents leaked out of the defect and caused severe sepsis. He underwent an operation which left him with a colostomy bag.

"Hi Bob. My name is Mark. I'm one of the doctors here. You might not remember, but I've been taking care of you for the last few days in ICU. How are you today?"

"Shh, quiet. Don't let them hear you," as he pointed at the nurses at the end of the bay, staring at them through wide, suspicious eyes. He then put his index finger again towards his lips and produced a long "shhhh".

"Why? What did they do?" I asked

"They're policewomen. Last night, they dragged me by the neck."

I realised he was referring to the line inserted in his neck. Bob had been put on renal replacement therapy, or a kidney machine, but the line kept obstructing with each neck movement overnight, so much so that the nurses had to constantly turn his head towards the left for the flow to be maintained.

"Bob, those are nurses. Remember you have a big line in your neck for the kidney machine. Do you know where you are?" I smiled as I pushed further.

"A sewer. Deep dark sewer. Lots of sewage around. It was blocked, and then sewage started leaking everywhere!"

He wasn't entirely wrong there, considering the amount of faecal contamination in his abdomen a few days prior. I had explained his operation several times over the last few days. But in his delirious state, Bob's mind conjured up a dramatic escape scene like that from a thriller movie. I couldn't help but laugh a little and noticed that the nurse standing by his bed was also sniggering. Somehow, finding amusement in such encounters allows us to cope with our inability to explain all that we see. In a bid to re-orientate Bob, I persisted in repeating where he was, what had happened, and who we were.

"Not quite Bob. You are on the Intensive Care Unit in Queen Elizabeth Hospital. It's the 24th of February 2024. You just had major surgery on your bowel. I can understand why you say that, but you are not in a sewer."

"Hmm, I feel a bit muddled at the moment."

"Yes, I think you might be a bit confused. Well, you are safe here on the ICU. The nurse looking after you is Leanne. You just have a little rest for the moment. We need to restart that kidney machine very soon," I said, pointing to the dialysis machine.

"You mean the children riding bicycles?"

"What children?"

"There," he pointed at the haemofiltration machine, "the wheels go round and round." He proceeded to draw circles in the air with his fingers.

"Ah yes, those are roller pumps. As they go around, the blood gets pumped from those lines in your neck. It then filters the blood and returns it." I tried to explain but only got a blank expression in return.

After a few days of re-orientation and recovery, Bob finally regained his cognition. Like many other patients suffering from delirium, he remembered part of his experiences as I spoke to him.

"I know you. You're the doctor who plays the bass," said Bob, referring to a conversation we had a couple of days prior. I had previously tried to find a common interest to exercise his memory, and found out that he played music in an amateur band, too.

"Yes, that's right, my name is Mark. I've been taking care of you for the last few days. Do you remember where you are and what has happened?" I asked, trying to test his recall.

He then told me of how he remembered being confused but couldn't quite work out what was happening. Able to receive sensory information but unable to process it correctly, Bob's perception of the circumstances was tempered by his professional training as a social worker. I was sure his mind was partially able to piece together what we said, even though he did not completely understand. He knew he was confused, and with regular reminders, he eventually picked up the fact that he was in a healthcare facility, being taken care of by doctors and nurses.

During the day, delirium is often considered a manageable inconvenience, a minor adverse effect of the critical illness. However, at night, the manifestations of delirium multiply in a phenomenon we colloquially term "sun-downing". The skeletal staffing, coupled with circadian biology, which we still do not fully comprehend, sometimes results in more dramatic situations.

Take bodybuilder Sam, for example, who was admitted to ICU after taking an overdose of heroin. Since heroin causes respiratory depression, he ended up being intubated to control his breathing. After he was extubated, he became delirious but seemed calm during the day. However, in the middle of the night, he jumped out of bed, ripped off his gown and stormed off the ICU. The nurse-in-charge tried to chase him but was afraid to confront his muscular, 6ft frame. So, she called security and alerted the ICU doctor-on-call, Sarah.

Sam wandered around the corridors surrounding the ICU, trying to open doors, clearly disoriented and confused. Before the security guards arrived, Sam had made his way into the staff room. Naked, with a catheter hanging out of his penis, he turned on the lights and stood in the doorway, giving the four nurses on their break a wakeup call they would never forget. Unable to escape, all they could do was scream at the sight, which they had no choice but to behold, waiting for the security guards to arrive.

The screaming nurses provoked Sam even more, who then shouted back. Fortunately, the doctor-on-call, Sarah, had arrived and called loudly to Sam before he could get any closer to the nurses. The security guards arrived, a short elderly gentleman and an equally small-statured young man. Sarah realised they would be no match for Sam's strength. She patiently explained the situation and place to Sam and very slowly, over ten minutes, managed to get close enough to inject a large dose of haloperidol into his central line, which soon calmed him down sufficiently to guide him back to his bed, where he then slept very soundly the rest of the night. The nurses, though, could not sleep after that.

Then, there was old granny Mary Smith, who was recovering well from her pneumonia, but one night decided all the staff were trying to kill her. At around midnight, she asked the nurse to help her to the toilet but then, once inside, got hold of the showerhead and used it as a weapon. She stood in the doorway and began wildly swinging the showerhead at whoever dared to approach.

"Mary, you're in hospital. Can you see our uniforms?" I pointed at the nurses and my own hospital scrubs. "These are nurses, and I'm the doctor taking care of you. You're in Queen Elizabeth Hospital in the intensive care unit. You are safe, and we are all looking after you."

This was my usual opening gambit – re-orientation to time, place, and person, emphasising safety and pointing out facts. Mary was having none of it.

"I don't believe you!" she scowled as she used the showerhead to point in our direction. "Liars, all of you! I'm calling the police! You stay away from me, all you bastards!" Her sweet, high-pitched voice stood in sharp contrast to the vulgar words she was shouting.

"No, Mary. Look around you... can you see all the other patients? Will you just put the showerhead down, at least? We don't want anyone to get hurt." I kept my hands at my side and in front of me, not wanting to be construed as hiding a weapon, so I thought. I turned my head to the nurse on my left and whispered, "Could you get some haloperidol, please?"

She nodded and went to fetch the tranquillisation drug.

"Don't you come any closer. I'll whack you; I'm telling you."

"Okay Mary, I believe you. But you're going to hurt yourself like that. Please put it down and come and sit down. We can give you a cup of tea if you want." I tried a different tack.

As I stood there, I noted the cannula in her left forearm. But there was no way to sneak up behind her to use it. Rushing in to restrain her was equally dangerous. Not only did we run the risk of causing her to fall and potentially fracture her hip, but any one of the staff members could also be injured by the bludgeon in her hand.

"No way. You all just want to kill me. Go away. I want to go home!" She cried.

The exchange went on for a further five minutes, during which I realised there was no way around this and whispered a plan to some of the nurses. Mary continued to wave the showerhead wildly, but as I walked to her left and kept her attention, I signalled to the nurse-in-charge, who then stood a metre from her right shoulder. She swiftly lunged towards Mary, grabbing the showerhead while two other nurses brought a chair in and wrestled her onto it. At the same time, I grabbed onto her left forearm with my left hand and quickly injected the syringe of haloperidol directly into the cannula. The struggling and screaming persisted for another minute while we waited for the drug to take its effect, after which we all heaved sighs of relief.

Night or day, a universal manifestation of delirium seems to be the desire for freedom from all foreign lines or objects. Patients may try to pull ECG electrodes, remove saturations probes, or – in many cases – climb out of bed. Many of these attempts are benign, but there are some which end a little more dramatically.

This was the case with Lisa. She was admitted after a gastrointestinal (GI) bleed from a stomach ulcer. She lost a tremendous amount of blood and required about 20 packs of various blood components during her four-hour emergency operation. After she was extubated, disoriented and withdrawn, she sat quietly in her bed. When the nurse came back from her toilet break, she pulled back the curtain to a disturbing sight. Lisa had pulled her arterial line out from her wrist, broken the stitches which held it onto her skin, and – in Golem-like fashion – sat hunched in bed, licking up each precious drop of blood from its tip. A blue-black bruise had begun to form on the wrist where the arterial line was inserted, and blood was slowly flowing onto the sheets. The nurse quickly removed the arterial line from her hands and put pressure on the wound while two other nurses began changing the sheets. Lisa did not remember her vampiric hunger after her delirium had resolved.

Then there was Harry, an elderly man who, in his confusion, became obsessed with the urinary catheter. He was caught many times playing with the latex tube hanging out of his penis, twirling it around his finger, tugging on it. This same genital obsession is not uncommon amongst young men and boys during emergence from anaesthesia, who immediately grab their crotches to check if they still possess their own penis. An extreme form even has its own recognised psychiatric diagnosis: "koro" or genital retraction syndrome.

This syndrome was originally described in Southeast Asia, where the Malay *koro* is translated as "to shrink", or *kura* is the word for the head of a tortoise, also a slang word for the penis. Harry continued tugging at his catheter till one day, lying in bed with his hands under the sheets, he managed to pull out the entire catheter, balloon still inflated, back out through his urethra, and out of his penis. The bloody mess was noticed quickly by the nurse, who saw the wet pink patch of blood mixed with urine in the middle of the sheets. Every male staff member cringed as they walked past and realised what had happened.

Amusing as some of these vignettes are, delirium is unfortunately not entirely benign. Up to a third of patients with critical-care-associated delirium go on to develop long-term cognitive impairment, like dementia. As such, ICUs around the world develop different methods to optimise environmental factors for the prevention of delirium. They aim to align the intensive care environment to normality, including low lighting at night, minimal disturbances of sleep if possible, empowering relatives to be involved in care, various communication aids, restoring day-night environments and maintaining oral nutrition if possible.

Intensive care follow-up clinics are offered in some units, attempting to reconcile some of the traumatic perceptions with explanations and explorations of patient journeys in intensive care. Through these clinics, psychological support is offered to ICU survivors to prevent or minimise post-traumatic disorders and severe mental health sequelae. But one does not need a medical degree to recognise the extreme circumstances patients face in ICU, nor to understand the potential for severe mental harm as a result. The visceral reactions of visiting relatives upon seeing their loved one discoloured, sedated, ventilated, penetrated and artificially kept alive, prove that torture is indeed easier to recognise than it is to define. Intensive care sometimes really seems like torture. But...

We will hold your hand and be your friend when you are isolated on the unit. We will speak when you can't and keep quiet when you need the rest. We will help you clean, shave, eat and drink. We will remind you of the day, time, and place, and we will return your autonomy as soon as we can. Maybe then, the

ICU may not be a place of torture, but one of rest, safety and recovery. Perhaps then, the worst scars may not be in the mind.

"Round like a circle in a spiral, like a wheel within a wheel
Never ending or beginning on an ever-spinning reel
As the images unwind, like the circles that you find
In the windmills of your mind!"
- Alan and Marilyn Bergman

17. Gymnopédie

Oblique et coupant l'ombre un torrent éclatant
Ruisselait en flots d'or sur la dalle polie
Où les atomes d'ambre au feu se miroitant
Mêlaient leur sarabande à la gymnopédie

Slanting and shadow-cutting a bursting stream
Trickled in gusts of gold on the shiny flagstone
Where the amber atoms in the fire gleaming
Mingled their sarabande with the gymnopaedia.

- J.P. Contamine de Latour

The Latin motto *"divinum sedare dolorem"*, translated as "it is divine to alleviate pain", is printed on the crest of the Royal College of Anaesthetists, leaving no doubt about a primary responsibility within the specialty of anaesthesia and intensive care.[36] Along with this motto, several key elements of analgesia are depicted within the shield on the crest. The poppy seedpod, from which morphine is extracted, features in the topmost band. Coca leaves, from which cocaine originates, lie in two quadrants of the shield, representing local anaesthesia.[37]

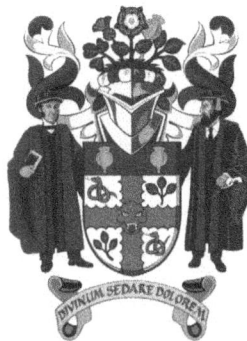

---

[36] The specialty of intensive care medicine originated from the work of anaesthetists. Indeed, many intensivists continue to also be anaesthetists.

[37] Boulton T. The College Crest London: Royal College of Anaesthetists; [Available from: https://rcoa.ac.uk/about-college/heritage/college-crest.]

These days, analgesia can be achieved using a wide variety of techniques. Commonly known are oral or injected medications, from simple paracetamol to anti-inflammatories and opioids. Minor surgery can be performed with local anaesthetics infiltrated into a small site, but knowledge of anatomy also allows us to block specific nerves for pain relief. For example, blocking the femoral and cutaneous nerve (called a fascia iliaca block) dramatically reduces the pain associated with a fractured hip.

Injecting local anaesthetic into the sheaths surrounding the intercostal nerves of the chest provides pain relief for rib fractures and allows patients to breathe effectively. Epidural analgesia, like those used in labour, can not only be used to augment the pain of childbirth but may also be used for performing a Caesarian section. Indeed, the crest encapsulates many of the agents we continue to rely on for analgesia these days. But to me, it still lacks a key instrument.

——●◆●——

Margaret was a frail old lady who had undergone a major abdominal operation to remove a large tumour in her colon. She came back to ICU with rectus sheath catheters. These two small catheters continually infused local anaesthetic around the nerves of the abdominal wall. However, this had failed to control her pain sufficiently. Over the course of the night, she groaned and writhed around in bed, so was given a Patient Controlled Analgesia (PCA) in addition. She pressed the button connected to the pump many times, which provided opioids directly into her veins every five minutes. While this alleviated some of her pain, she still looked miserable during the morning ward round. Her eyebrows continued to be furrowed. Her breaths were shallow, and she sat perfectly still in bed for fear of precipitating more pain. We were concerned that with such suboptimal analgesia, she would develop a chest infection. I urged her to take deep breaths. I threatened her with the complications of pneumonia. I sent the physiotherapists to work with her. Despite all of these, Margaret continued to take shallow breaths and cough ineffectively due to her pain.

Guitarist Leigh was a regular volunteer at the ICU. She was dressed in a black turtleneck sweater, a tartan-style knee-length pleated skirt and bright pink tights, which extended into her black patent Dr. Martens boots. Her purple sling held her guitar high on her chest. Her blond hair had purple-coloured tips and was tied in a messy ponytail. Such "unprofessional" attire would not have complied with any hospital uniform policy. It was indeed a stark departure from the robes of the Royal College of Physicians and Surgeons worn by John Snow and Joseph Clover, respectively, distinguished supporters of the shield of the Royal College of Anaesthetists. A nurse or doctor dressed in a fashion like Leigh would have been reprimanded and asked to change immediately. Yet, Leigh provided relief beyond the limits of medical science. But I was not surprised.

Bound by the assumed expectations of patients, healthcare professionals are regularly told to "dress conservatively" so as not to cause offence. We were encouraged for some time to even skirt around words like "dying" so as not to cause distress (this sometimes backfired, for the vague alternative terms – like "deteriorating" or "not doing too well" – failed to address the key fear of patients and their relatives: death). Much like the reductionist approach to medicine and a heavily biomedical view of health, we oftentimes fail to consider wider aspects of holistic wellbeing. But why should we be bland when our work is one of emotional extremes? Why should we look unfashionable when we are required to keep up to date with the latest scientific progress? Why should we pride ourselves on being "business-like" when our patients yearn for a personal approach?

Anatole Broyard quotes a "lack of style or magic" as the basis for his lack of trust in a particular doctor in his essay *The Patient Examines the Doctor*. The universal white theatre cap failed to speak to his character. The use of scientific vocabulary without poetic application failed to touch his soul. The utilitarianism of the hospital and its staff failed to capture the beauty of his spirit. He, like many patients, especially those who are critically ill, yearns not just for a cure, but an easing of suffering, one which can be facilitated only through a trusting doctor-patient relationship.

My wife once wore to her clinic a matching opal necklace and earrings set we bought together in Australia. Such jewellery was strongly discouraged in her hospital. The patient, Sarah, a young and anxious jeweller who had cancer, noticed the colourful opal. This created a spark for a personal conversation about her work, her journey, and her intense fears regarding the operation. It created an opportunity for my wife to explain the operation not purely in technical terms but to hold an honest conversation about the risks, benefits, and personal choice. Sarah was so thankful for such a connection that she wanted my wife to perform the operation, even though she was just the junior surgeon at that stage.

Similarly, both my wife and I have a selection of colourful surgical caps we wear into theatre. I wear them despite some hospitals prohibiting the use of personal surgical caps. One of my favourites is made from a print of many different cartoon dinosaurs. We bought this fabric from a backstreet store in Singapore, the year before we got married. I have used this on many occasions to gain the trust of children needing emergency operations. Those magical creatures have allowed me to calm many screams, disarm many defences, and explain our techniques and equipment using concepts which interest young minds.

My wife's opals and my dinosaur scrub cap are but some of the "magic" required to reach through the facade of biomedicine into the heart of suffering and fear. Being part of our journey and narrative, such items let patients into our own personal stories, shared experiences, joys and fears. It forms landmarks and signposts for our patients' own journeys and narratives, far more so than the solid-coloured dress shirt and dark trousers of many doctors' dress codes or the opaque black tights required underneath nurses' uniforms.

I was glad that the ridiculous rules surrounding attire in hospitals did not extend to volunteer musicians. If medicine can be considered the artistic application of science, then we should return the individuality and personality of healthcare professionals. And it could perhaps begin with what we wear.

Leigh started playing her guitar outside the double doors leading into the first bay of four female patients. I recognised it immediately as Erik Satie's *Gymnopédie*. Widely regarded as one of the most relaxing pieces of music in history, one wouldn't guess it from the musical directions of *Lent et douloureux* (slow and painfully) written at the start of the piece. Accordingly, Satie's rise to musical fame was equally troubled and tortuous. Born in Normandy in 1866, Satie started learning the piano at the age of six. In 1882, his initial hopes of musical fame were dashed when he failed to meet standards and was expelled three years after enrolling in the Paris Conservatory. Following this failure, Satie was again discharged for malingering after only a few months of military service. Deemed "untalented" and "lazy" by his tutors and superiors, Satie's early music career took a divergent direction to his close friend Claude Debussy, despite their common bohemian lifestyles.

Instead of the romantic and lyrical compositions that Debussy was so well-known for, many of Satie's pieces focused on unconventional and repetitive sounds. The use of propellers and sirens for his ballet *Parade* understandably failed to impress audiences who had recently been through the horrors of World War I. But despite his unconventional approach and rejection by his early contemporaries, Satie's contribution to music cannot be understated. Many of his later works were pivotal to the departure from French Romanticism and heavily influenced the minimalist movement of the 1950s.

Satie wrote *Gymnopédies* in 1888, soon after meeting the fellow Bohemian and poet Contamine de Latour. The French *gymnopédie* is seen in music dictionaries as a nude dance by young Spartan maidens accompanied by song. This is further traced back to the Greek *gymnopaedia*, an annual festival of naked (or unarmed) young men dancing. Ironically, the *douloureux* in the musical directions possesses the same root as the Latin *dolorem* from the crest of the Royal College of Anaesthetists above, the same pain it would soon divinely alleviate. The piece began slowly and regularly, centred around two repetitive major seventh chords, with a rhythmically unexciting, occasionally dissonant melody which frequently resolves within short phrases.

As Leigh played, she walked into the middle of the bay, each step deliberate – as calculated and predictable as the accompaniment. Yet there was a spring and a sway in her step – the coyness of musical tension. Leigh faced Margaret in bed two, and – with a demure smile – invited her to join in their own imaginary *gymnopédie* dance.

Leigh's and Margaret's eyes engaged. Margaret nodded to imply consent. Through music, they were transported beyond the confines of the ICU. The connection was intense and intimate, like a slow dance on a fine sandy beach. Within their imaginary embrace, Margaret was comforted by the regular rhythm and the open harmonies, much like how one allows oneself to enjoy the constant heartbeat and slow breaths of a partner. For those two minutes, she existed beyond the pain of a 20-centimetre midline laparotomy wound, breathing deep, slow breaths which her pain had not allowed just a few minutes earlier. Now, during their *gymnopédie,* she seemed to inhale the fragrance of the sea rather than the ICU odours of faeces and chlorine. She waved her arms with the music, imagining the excitement of each swing, turn and pirouette. The heady feeling after a good spin remained as Leigh slowly made her way around the bay.

The effect was reproducible in bed three, and again in bed four. Even more amazingly, it was not confined to the patients. The entire unit seemed to suddenly slow down. Staff conversation turned from complaining about daily grievances to chatting about enjoying music, from their favourite artistes to the latest musicals they had watched. With Leigh's presence and music, the ICU bay became a seaside lounge. The regular beeping of the monitors were waves rolling up on the shore. The bright medical lights, a surrogate for the warming rays of the sun. The morphine used in many of our patients could well have passed for strong ouzo, completing the picture of a *gymnopédie* on a sunny Greek beach.

Through processes not entirely understood, music alters not only emotional states but accelerates healing processes and complements many aspects of medicine. Pain relief and relaxation through music have been demonstrated in several scientific studies and reviews.[38,39] The ancient Greek mathematician Pythagoras observed the emotional catharsis that occurs with music. Likewise, Plato recognised the power of music as a way of conditioning and curing the soul, which in his philosophy was intricately linked to the body. To him, music encompassed vocal and instrumental sound production, as well as body movements and dance. Indeed, music therapy has been used in many branches of medicine for different benefits and to various degrees. Music has been shown to reduce pain and opioid use in intensive care, improve symptoms of neuromuscular and psychiatric disorders,[40] and benefit social functioning for people with autism.[41] Similarly, dance has been shown to improve cognitive function, delay the progression of neuropsychiatric disorders,[42] and aid in coping mechanisms for chronic diseases.[43] All these studies report minimal to no side effects – a finding that is virtually impossible with pharmacological agents and drugs.

From anxiolysis and analgesia to channelling hope and "soul medicine",[44] music therapy fills a gap which medical practice

[38] Umbrello M, Sorrenti T, Mistraletti G, Formenti P, Chiumello D, Terzoni S. Music therapy reduces stress and anxiety in critically ill patients: a systematic review of randomized clinical trials. Minerva Anestesiol. 2019;85(8):886-98.

[39] Richard-Lalonde M, Gélinas C, Boitor M, Gosselin E, Feeley N, Cossette S, et al. The Effect of Music on Pain in the Adult Intensive Care Unit: A Systematic Review of Randomized Controlled Trials. J Pain Symptom Manage. 2020;59(6):1304-19.e6.

[40] Kamioka H, Tsutani K, Yamada M, Park H, Okuizumi H, Tsuruoka K, et al. Effectiveness of music therapy: a summary of systematic reviews based on randomized controlled trials of music interventions. Patient Prefer Adherence. 2014;8:727-54.

[41] Geretsegger M, Fusar-Poli L, Elefant C, Mossler KA, Vitale G, Gold C. Music therapy for autistic people. Cochrane Database Syst Rev. 2022;5(5):CD004381.

[42] Li K, Weng L, Wang X. The State of Music Therapy Studies in the Past 20 Years: A Bibliometric Analysis. Front Psychol. 2021;12:697726.

[43] Strassel JK, Cherkin DC, Steuten L, Sherman KJ, Vrijhoef HJ. A systematic review of the evidence for the effectiveness of dance therapy. Altern Ther Health Med. 2011;17(3):50-9.

[44] Schiffman R. The Healing Power of Music New York: New York Times; 2021 [Available from: https://www.nytimes.com/2021/04/08/well/music-therapy-treatment-stress.html.

cannot. From the claustrophobic confines of the ICU to the expanse of a Greek beach, the imaginations of both patients and staff were caught that afternoon.

I should have known.

I have experienced the euphoria of many musical climaxes during my previous orchestral performances. I have witnessed the rapture in the faces of audiences at the end of a piece. I have seen the way music can channel and direct emotions.

I should not have been surprised.

Throughout history, music has been used in conjunction with healing. Ancient Egyptian frescoes depicted the use of music within healing rites from about 4,000 BCE. The *Bimarhane* hospital in the ancient Turkish city of Amasya regularly used music as part of their treatment regimes in the 1300s CE.[45] The Chinese idiom 樂先藥後 demonstrates a clear linguistic link between music and medicine. Directly translated, it means "music first, medicine after" or "music before medicine". The characters are displayed in traditional script (樂先藥後) rather than the more modern simplified script of 乐先药后. This is because, in the former, the character for music (樂) is almost identical to the character for medicine (藥) except for the heading (or grass radical), which denotes that medicine has plant or herbal origins. The ancient Greeks similarly attributed both healing and music to a single deity: Apollo. For generations, his name was invoked during graduations from medical school as the preamble to the Hippocratic Oath:

"I swear by Apollo physician, by Asclepius, by Hygeia, by Panacea, and by all the gods and goddesses, making them my witnesses, that I will carry out, according to my ability and judgment, this oath and this indenture."

Clearly, the ancient Greeks believed that Apollo was not the only deity with healing powers. The inclusion of Apollo's son Asclepius, as well as Asclepius' daughters within the Oath, reflected their understanding of the complex and multi-faceted healing journey. Asclepius himself was regarded as the god of

---

[45] Sandlow LJ. The hospital that treated patients with music. Hektoen International. 2020;12(4).

medicine. Asclepius' daughters continue to personify many aspects of modern medicine. Hygeia (Hygiene) and Panacea (Universal remedy) were two obvious mentions within the Hippocratic Oath. However, Asclepius had three other daughters: Iaso (recuperation), Acceso (healing process) and Aegle (glow of health). But what of Apollo's other major attribute: music? Apollo was also credited with the creation of the lyre, an instrument regarded by the ancient Greeks as producing the most beautiful sounds. Like a harp, Apollo's lyre would have consisted of taut strings around a U-shaped frame. But it is also usually portrayed with a small sound box, not unlike that of Leigh's guitar.

The synergism between the various members of the ICU team was crucial to Margaret's recovery journey. The drugs of Panacea (universal remedy) provided life support. Iaso (recuperation) was delivered through rest and compassionate nursing. Hygeia (hygiene), as promoted by the clean habits of the ICU, helped prevent further infections and complications. The "healing process" of Aceso was accelerated through good physiotherapy and nutrition. But the cold, unfamiliar and utilitarian ICU environment and the bland, unflattering, and unfashionable uniforms of the staff arguably failed to achieve the *glow of health* in her, as much as we tried. In the end, it was the invocation of music which promoted the holistic healing required for Margaret to progress through her recovery journey. So, with music ringing in her ears, and as their *gymnopédie* drew to a close, Margaret was left with the naked glow of Aegle (glow of health). Typhon, the beast of human affliction throughout Greek mythology, during those minutes of gymnopédie, was utterly defeated by the lyre of Apollo, or in this case, the guitar of Leigh.

"Now then, putrefy here on the earth which nourishes people! Nor will you live any more as an evil affliction to mortals…" - Hymn for Apollo (translated by Rodney Merrill)

[2nd prize winner for the Health Education England essay competition 2021. An extract was originally published by Intensive Care Medicine journal and was their top social media impact piece of their *From the Inside* section in 2022. Tan MZY. Gymnopédie: music in the ICU. Intensive Care Medicine (Springer Nature). 2023;49(2):267-8. Available from: [https://link.springer.com/article/10.1007/s00134-022-06935-3] Used with permission.]

18. 求签
Chinese Fortune Sticks

"For even the very wise cannot see all ends."
- J.R.R Tolkien, The Fellowship of the Ring

Schick schick schick schick clickety clack.

A single chopstick falls out from the wooden container. Chosen, as if by luck. On it, a Chinese number. The smell of incense fills the courtyard, and the large brass urn frames the other worshippers. Knelt on mats, each of them holds an identical container with about 30 chopsticks inside. The containers are shaken. Their heads are bowed. Their mouths mutter prayers. In front of them sits a statue of Buddha. He is gold. His legs are crossed. His left hand rests on his lap, palm facing up as if holding the entire world within its grasp. His right hand is held in front of his chest, fingers extended in a praying form. The worshippers present their requests and prayers to him and seek answers within those chopsticks.

Schick schick schick schick schick clickety clack. 四 *(sì). The number four.*

The number four, in Mandarin Chinese, but more particularly in the Hokkien dialect, are all homonyms of the word 死 *(si):* to die. They all sound similar and are considered bad luck. £4 or £40 are never given as gifts for weddings or occasions. No gift should contain the number four. It is inauspicious. Four foretells unfavourable fortune.

The number eight (八), on the other hand, is the opposite. It is a homonym of 发 *(fa),* particularly in the Cantonese dialect. 发财 *(fa cai)* describes getting rich. So, the red packets given as Chinese New Year gifts from elders to children of the extended family often contain £8, and red packets used as wedding gifts frequently contain £88.

I was only a child when the chopstick with "四" dropped out of my auntie's wooden container. I was sometimes taken along to these temple visits, even though my immediate family is Christian. Such is the testament to Singapore's commitment to multi-religiousness. I have visited Buddhist and Hindu temples, witnessed the ceremonies of all four major religions, and visited friends during their respective celebrations. But while I shared in the festivities, I reserved my judgment for some of the beliefs. In this case, I cared little for the divination practice of shaking chopsticks.

I remember looking into divination as a teenager and learning about the ancient Mesopotamian practice of observing flickering flames or animal entrails and telling someone's fortune. It seemed ridiculous. I also remember another example when learning about beekeeping. Some beekeepers use dowsing when deciding where to place their beehives. Even medical botanist and conservationist Dr Diana Beresford-Kroeger wrote about getting a local dowser to locate a good water source for digging a well in her Canadian farm. Dowsing involves loosely holding a bent copper rod (or other sticks) in each hand and walking around. The movements of the copper rods signify invisible forces, and when the rods cross each other, it suggests either a meeting of those forces or buried objects in the ground. The beekeepers justify it with anecdotal experience of some honeybee colonies building messy honeycombs across several empty frames. When they shifted the orientation of the hive based on dowsing, the cross-comb stopped, and the bees somehow then built their combs nicely within the frames provided. I thought it was completely bonkers, but soon learnt even large utility companies in the UK continued to use it well into the 21st century. I'm still not sure I buy it.

My auntie, seemingly through bad luck, managed to pick the chopstick with number four written on it. She took it to the priest, fearing the worst. The priest took the chopstick and referred to his almanac. It contained a collection of idioms and cryptic phrases that changed according to several variables, including the date and time. Fortunately, there weren't any predictions of my auntie's death. Instead, the priest said that my auntie would experience family struggles that year. The struggles were a test of her faith, but she would overcome them. I guess it was a sufficiently generic statement to believe in.

Schick schick schick schick clickety clack

In medicine, we like to think we have better methods than shaking chopsticks or looking into crystal balls. We instead use the term "prognostication". Prognostication describes the practice of predicting recovery or deterioration. It formed a key distinguishing feature of the ancient Hippocratic physicians and galvanised the observational approach to science and medicine.

Based on the observation of certain constellations of symptoms or signs, physicians could predict health outcomes, enabling patients to be prepared for the likely trajectories of their illnesses. As time went on, our ways of prognosticating became more sophisticated. Today, the modern physician may use many methods to help them predict a patient's outcome. These may include history and examination, simple blood tests, radiological imaging, physiological function tests, body tissue samples and large datasets.

For many diseases and conditions, we can prognosticate with a high level of certainty. Through history and examination, we can tell the severity of a failing heart. Using various investigations, we have highly validated five-year survival statistics on many types of cancers. We can quite accurately predict death within a few days after a cardiac arrest from radiological imaging and physical signs. We learn very quickly as junior doctors to identify the sick-looking patients for referral to intensive care. Yet there are almost no tests which are 100% accurate, and no prognostic method which provides full certainty that a patient will recover or die. Our measurements and metrics, in which we put our faith, sometimes deceive us. Many intensivists will have their own stories of patients who have surprised entire teams, making miraculous recoveries despite being given poor prognoses. Many doctors have similar tales of patients who have far surpassed their predictions of deterioration and death.

———◆◆———

Schick schick schick schick clickety clack

Bert lay in a bed on the intensive care unit. Opposite him on the other side of the unit lay Cher, both in equally bad states. They were both intubated and ventilated. They had both been in the intensive care unit for at least five days with unclear diagnoses.

Bert, a man in his seventies, was admitted to hospital after his wife found him drowsy and less responsive than usual. A month prior to this episode, he had had a transient ischaemic attack: a mini-stroke. He made a good recovery from this. But on this episode, he was so drowsy that he could not clear his own saliva. Each time he breathed, he gurgled. I imagined saliva dripping down his trachea, flowing into the right lung, clogging it up and brewing a chest infection. We had to intubate him to prevent this from happening. He was then put on a ventilator. He was also experiencing seizures, and we had to start anti-epileptic medications.

Initial investigations were inconclusive. A CT scan of his head did not show any obvious diagnosis, and blood tests were almost normal. We performed a lumbar puncture. The cerebrospinal fluid obtained from this was completely normal. After almost a week of daily turning off his sedation to test his neurological status, he remained too drowsy to breathe adequately for himself. He would take a breath only every ten seconds or so, clearly insufficient to maintain life. The only other response we could elicit from him was a flicker of movement in his shoulders each time we put a long suction tube inside his windpipe (or trachea) to clear his secretions. There was not even a cough reflex on irritation of his airway.

An electroencephalogram (EEG) was done. This tracing of the electrical activity of the brain involved multiple electrode pads placed on various points on the head. An analysis of the trace showed diffuse encephalopathy, a non-specific sign of brain dysfunction associated with a poor prognosis. A CT scan of the brain also failed to show any reversible causes of his drowsiness. All the tests we performed pointed us to a poor prognosis. We prepared ourselves to withdraw life support on him and allow him to die.

Schick schick schick schick schick clickety clack. 四 *(sì). The number four.*

Cher was about 20 years younger than Bert. She, too, had had a stroke a month prior to this episode. The first time I met her, she was already sedated on a breathing machine. She was initially found slumped in her bedroom, body sprawled half on the bed and half upon the windowsill. She was blue, a manifestation of the low oxygen levels in her blood. Her carers commenced cardiopulmonary resuscitation (CPR) while calling the ambulance. It was unclear if she had had a heart attack, but when the paramedics arrived, she certainly needed help with her breathing, even if not her heart. Cher's daughter had arrived at that time and pointed the crew to the empty blister packs of codeine and diazepam close to the bed. It had transpired that Cher had been addicted to prescription drugs for over a year before this episode, and it was likely that she had taken an overdose of these drugs the day before. The codeine especially would have caused her respiratory rate to slow down and blunted the body's normal responses to low oxygen and high carbon dioxide.

We spent the first few days of Cher's stay correcting some electrolytes and allowing her body to metabolise the drugs she had taken. She was ventilated as she initially made little effort to breathe. She was also sedated to help her tolerate being on a ventilator. Several days later, we were still unable to extubate Cher. Each time we turned the sedation off, she stared into space and produced no meaningful responses to our shouts or shakes. By this time, the drugs would have been metabolised and cleared by the body, but she was still unresponsive. We ordered a repeat CT scan. It did not show anything new. We called the neurologist. He came to assess both Cher and Bert.

"They both show signs of severe brain damage. At best, they might be in a persistent vegetative state," he said.

Schick schick schick schick schick clickety clack. 四 (sì). The number four again.

The next day, we escorted Bert for an MRI head scan. We had booked it prior, and the neurologist had mentioned it would be helpful in prognostication to look for small areas of brain damage. The plan was to complete the MRI, hold a final discussion between the team and the family, and then withdraw life support to let him die. We prepared the family and called the specialist neuroradiologist and the neurologist. I then made my way with Bert's nurse and a porter down to the MRI scanner. Since the entire trip took over two hours, I knew it would be time for me to hand over to the night team upon my return. But as I entered the MRI scanning room to transfer Bert back onto his bed, he started to cough on the breathing tube. This was new. He was not able to do this before. I thought little of it, but he started doing it again on the way back to ICU. By the time we made it through the long corridor, up the lift and round the bend to ICU, Bert had started taking some breaths on the ventilator. Again, this was an improvement. We parked him in his bed space, reconnected the infusions and monitors, and changed over the ventilator. And then I noticed a flicker in his little finger on his right hand. Within the next hour, Bert's hand had begun to reach for the breathing tube. But it was time for me to hand over.

"Bed five, Bert. Presumed hypoxic brain injury. Poor prognosis confirmed by neurologists. He had his MRI scan this afternoon with a view to withdraw care after, but he has started to show purposeful movements," I presented.

There were a few exclamations of surprise and faces of shock from the night team.

"I know," I resumed, "it's almost as if the MRI has aligned all his brain cells again!" I joked, referring to the incredibly strong magnets of the MRI machine.

There were a few nervous sniggers. We became slightly uncomfortable that we were prepared to withdraw life support on him just hours ago.

The next day was Friday. Bert had regained sufficient muscle power to tug at the breathing tube. We asked him to open his eyes. He did. We asked if he wanted the tube out. He nodded. We removed it, and he was wide awake. We could not explain it, and neither could the MRI, CT, EEG, or blood tests. At the opposite end of the ICU, Cher also started to wake up. Like Bert, she too opened her eyes on command and nodded to our questions. She, too, was extubated that Friday.

Schick schick schick schick clickety clack. 八 (bā) The number eight.

Did Bert have a stroke? Unlikely. Did he attempt suicide with drugs? Perhaps. Was his brain damaged? Almost certainly, even if invisibly so. Did Cher suffer hypoxic brain injury? Possibly. Could the drugs have been in her body for longer than expected? Perhaps. Did we have sufficient information to withdraw life support? Yes, generally. Were we wrong to think about withdrawal? No, I don't think so. Why, then, did they both recover? I don't know. Will this affect my future practice? Quite probably.

There is a Chinese classical epic called Journey to the West (西游记). In one story, the monkey god, Sun Wu Kong (孙悟空), tries to usurp the position of the Jade Emperor of heaven (玉皇大帝). The commotion is eventually stopped by Buddha, who challenges Sun Wu Kong to escape his hand. If he could escape, Buddha would give him the title of Jade Emperor. Sun Wu Kong jumps on a cloud and travels to a distant land. As he turns to look back, he sees Buddha disappear in the distance and hears a faint laugh. He travels to a distant mountain range before deciding that he has succeeded in his task. But to prove it, he carves onto the mountain, "Sun Wu Kong was here", and then proceeds to urinate on the base of the mountain. After which, he flies back to Buddha, content and expectant.

"I have succeeded and flown to Five Peak Mountain. Go and see that I have left my mark, and then give me my crown," Sun Wu Kong says.

"I don't have to," replies Buddha, opening his palm, "look closely in my hand."

There on Buddha's ring finger was a small scribble with Sun Wu Kong's name.

"Smell it," Buddha went on.

Sun Wu Kong caught a whiff of urine and knew that he had not managed to escape Buddha's palm. He had failed. He had gained immortality, killed demons, and wrecked heaven, but he could not escape his fate, and when he tried to run away after this blunder, Buddha quickly turned his palm around and trapped Sun Wu Kong under Five Peak Mountain for 500 years.

Schick schick schick schick clickety clack

Like Sun Wu Kong's unescapable fate, Chinese fortune sticks, depending on the predisposition of the believer, carry a certain weight of destiny. But to the outsider, like my teenage self, focused on the sometimes reductionist explanations of science, such practices seem far-fetched. A few days later, I stood in the bay. Bert lay in a bed on the ICU, soundly sleeping. Opposite him on the other side of the unit lay Cher, this time watching television and gobbling down her lunch. Both equally alive. Two people with Lazarus revivals, narrowly escaping our hubris. Despite our sophisticated methods, we were unable to correctly predict their courses. It seemed we were no further along than shaking chopsticks in a bottle. When will they return to Buddha's palm? Only time will tell.

Postscript

The withdrawal of life support is a decision not made lightly. Yet, it occurs frequently within ICU. There is a perception that withdrawal of life support is synonymous with "giving up". This is not the case since many patients who come to ICU already have poor functional baselines. They have many co-morbidities, struggle to cope with daily activities, or have been deteriorating for months or years prior. In addition, there is often an unrealistic perception of what it means to survive ICU. Recovery from critical illness is often fraught with setbacks, complications and turmoil. ICU survivors may suffer from a host of complications. Up to 60% will experience mental health issues. 40% require physical rehabilitation. 33% never return to work. Without a robust network of support (whether family, friends or others), some survivors never achieve a quality of life that they are satisfied with. Having said that, when interviewed, many survivors are thankful for how intensive care saved their lives and would go through the experience again.

When we attempt to prognosticate, it is not purely a binary decision between life and death. While death may be a definite entity, life is a continuum which may extend from the nubile youth enjoying life to the chronically ill wishing they were dead. Ethical issues are countless even during the decision to admit to ICU. Intensivists question the likelihood of survival and the ability to recover against the knowledge of what most people want as a "good death", the numerous scoring systems available to predict mortality, the social determinants which affect potential recovery, and the clinical situation at hand. All this with very little information and limited time. By speaking to relatives or the patient themselves, if possible, we collect valuable pieces of a puzzle, attempting to gain insight into the patient's priorities and wishes. Integrating all this information helps us carefully tread the balance between allowing people to die and trying to save their lives. We do not always get it right.

Exposure

19. Grace

"Of all the forms of inequality, injustice in health care is the most shocking and inhumane." - Martin Luther King Jr

Mount Hagen is Papua New Guinea's third-largest city, with just over 45,000 people. I was stationed there in a small mission hospital on an elective placement just after qualifying from medical school. Seventeen-year-old Mercy was brought in by her friends, unresponsive, after a collapse. A CT head scan was needed, but there was no CT scanner. A lumbar puncture (LP) was performed instead. This would at least give us some information in the absence of the CT scan. When my needle penetrated the spinal canal, the cerebrospinal fluid (CSF) that flowed out was mixed with a bit of fresh blood. My needle could have hit a blood vessel on the way in, or so I thought. The lab analysis of the CSF was otherwise completely normal.

Mercy made a seemingly full recovery within 24 hours, only to experience another collapse a day later. This time, with her right pupil fixed and dilated, and clear neurological signs, the diagnosis became clear: she had had a subarachnoid haemorrhage. A sudden bleed into her brain – a catastrophic one. The blood I saw in the CSF was an initial "herald bleed", a warning sign for this larger, fatal bleed. Without a CT, no available neurosurgeon or interventional radiologist, and unable to fly to the capital for those services, she was doomed.

That night, I was called by the nurses to attend to five-month-old baby Grace, who was struggling to breathe. She had severe pneumonia and was already on the maximum flow of oxygen available there: a mere two litres per minute. This was less than a tenth of the flow rates found in most UK hospitals. Nebulisers and antibiotics were given, but despite this, her respiratory rate remained alarmingly high at 60 breaths per minute. Then, everything stopped. Respiratory arrest. The nurses scrambled to find a bag-valve-mask for me to ventilate. Too late. Her heart stopped. CPR started. I intubated. They finally got me a self-inflating bag. I stood there, forcing air (with the measly supplemental oxygen attached) into her lungs. This, together with CPR, restarted her heart.

For a moment, I had saved this baby's life. But then, I realised there were no ventilators in the hospital nor infusion pumps for sedation drugs. Grace, by now awake, had a plastic tube in her trachea and was forced to breathe with each squeeze of my hand. The mother, overwhelmed by the scene, silently stood beside the bed. My bleep went off. I was called to A&E for another emergency. As the only doctor in the hospital that night, I was left with little choice. I instructed the nurse to ventilate the baby and left. About an hour later, when I was on my way back from A&E, I heard the howls. Spine-shivering, toe-curling howls. Unmistakable sounds of a grieving mother. Grace had died. When I returned, I said very little. No words would have comforted her mother. I simply stood by the bedside with my hand on her mother's shoulder. I still shudder today when I recall the sound. Without the ability to provide basic critical care, it was near impossible for her to survive.

———◆◆———

Southwest Uganda. A district general hospital. The wards are bustling. Carers set up mattresses alongside the beds of their patients. Many of these carers are relatives of the patient. Without them, patients would have no providence for food or drink. Like a party, the wards ring with the chatter of patients and relatives, masking the occasional groans of suffering.

Strung across the staff room is what looks like bunting. On closer inspection, they are examination gloves that have been washed and are hanging up to dry for reuse. Blood products are frequently out of stock, oxygen is limited, and drugs are in short supply. That night, a young man named Nathaniel is brought into hospital after a car crash. Unlike the hospital in Papua New Guinea, this hospital had a CT scanner. Nathaniel's spleen has ruptured. It needs to be removed, but the hospital has no suitable sutures. The surgeons and I wait as the family scramble to the pharmacy down the road. They are closed, but the family's shouts have woken the owners of the pharmacy, who open the store and sell them the required sutures, which would enable the surgeons to close the wound after the operation.

Meanwhile, Nathaniel groans in pain as he continues to bleed from his spleen. We provide some oxygen and fluids. Then we wait. I get anxious, unaccustomed to the delay in life-saving treatment. An hour or so later, Nathaniel's family return to the hospital panting, bringing back the vital sutures needed to proceed with the operation. That night, the surgeons perform a splenectomy and save Nathaniel's life.

━━◆◆◆━━

What a contrast from the COVID-19 response in higher-income countries.

It took under two weeks for Chinese authorities to build and set up a 10,000-bed hospital in Wuhan. It took just nine days for the 4,000-bed London Nightingale Hospital to be prepared to receive critically ill COVID-19 patients. Ventilators by Dyson, hand gel from Louis Vuitton, 3D-printed equipment to keep healthcare workers safe. A stunning display of healthcare capacity amongst high-income countries. Yet, the strong undercurrents of global disparities barely featured in major news outlets. The Ethiopian prime minister implored higher-income nations to mount a global response to COVID-19, clearly worried about the impact of such a pandemic in lower-income countries where capacity is poor.

"Health for all" was the aim of the Alma Ata Declaration in 1978. Adopted by the World Health Organisation shortly after, this ambitious commitment sought to improve the healthcare systems by providing a common goal of accessible primary health care. Yet, over 40 years down the line, "Health for all" has failed to materialise.[46] Many countries still do not have access to primary health care. Many countries still do not have suitable equipment or expertise to manage critically ill patients.[47]

In 1948, after the destruction of vital infrastructure due to World War II, the UK government was keen to re-establish economic growth and stability. The needs of war had already accelerated the development of emergency medical services, but

---

[46] Hall JJ, Taylor R. Health for all beyond 2000: the demise of the Alma-Ata Declaration and primary health care in developing countries. Med J Aust. 2003;178:17-20.

[47] Baker T. Critical care in low-income countries. Tropical Medicine & International Health. 2009;14(2):143-8.

many hospitals were still private organisations serving the paying customer rather than the poor who would not have been able to afford medical care. Revolution arrived on the 5th of July 1948.[48] On that day, one of the most powerful lines of the then-Minister of Health, Aneurin Bevan, was contained within the opening statement of the newly launched National Health Service, "Everyone – rich or poor, man, woman or child – can use it or any part of it. There are no charges…"

The concept of grace resonates strongly and proudly in these lines from the NHS. Many people consider the UK's National Health Service (NHS) to be one of the first examples of socialised medicine. However, one of the earliest examples of charitable medical care was that provided for Egyptian workmen in Deir al-Medina in 1500 BCE. Workers in that city were not only provided with sick days but also had free access to a physician, which was no doubt a luxury service during that time.

By the time of the Byzantine Empire in c330 AD, establishments known as *nosokomia* (places of care) had sprouted across the empire, directly influenced by Christianity's teachings of grace and love for the less privileged. These *nosokomia* provided free medical care for the sick, in direct contrast to the prevailing practices at that time. This same commitment to universal healthcare was also found amongst the Islamic and Arab regions by the 1300s CE. Waqf charitable trust documents specifically allowed any patient, regardless of race, language, religion or economic status, to use the services of their *bimaristans* (hospitals).[49]

Back in the UK, I compare my experiences with those in Papua New Guinea and Uganda. When Pamela, a young and otherwise fit lady, collapsed while having dinner with friends, paramedics arrived within 20 minutes. She was assessed immediately upon arrival to A&E and got a CT scan within an hour. It showed a subarachnoid haemorrhage – the same condition young Mercy had had in Papua New Guinea.

---

[48] Tan MZY. 1948 healthcare: still appropriate today? Journal of the Royal Society of Medicine. 2023;0(0):01410768231214336.

[49] Pormann PE. 1001 Cures: Contributions in Medicine and Healthcare from Muslim Civilisation. Manchester: Foundation for Science Technology and Civilisation; 2018.

Neurosurgeons operated on her that night, and after several weeks in ICU, she recovered and was discharged home. Likewise, I remember seeing a six-month-old boy with severe pneumonia in A&E. Unlike little Grace in Papua New Guinea, he received high-flow nasal oxygen immediately. When he continued to deteriorate and suffer a cardiac arrest, several teams of specialists arrived within a minute. The A&E doctors and nurses took over CPR. I intubated him. He was put onto a ventilator while two other paediatricians inserted more IV lines for medications. Still, another doctor was already on the phone with the paediatric ICU team. He spent a further two days in the paediatric ICU before sadly dying, despite all the interventions.

I have also taken care of many trauma patients in the UK. Unlike Nathaniel in Uganda, there are never questions about the cost of life-saving emergency operations. Even barely mobile elderly patients who break their hip get it fixed within 36 hours of admission to hospital, because it dramatically reduces pain. Close to 80,000 hip fractures occur in the UK per year, and the vast majority are operated on.[50] The cost of each operation is estimated at £5,000 (USD $6,000) – about ten times the average annual income in Uganda, or twice that in Papua New Guinea.

Yes, there are huge global disparities in the availability, quality and accessibility of healthcare. But one patient really tested my faith in universal healthcare. Bruce was only 20 years old when he was first arrested. He ended up in prison several times for various crimes, but in this episode, he assaulted his girlfriend. The neighbours called the police. When they arrived, Bruce sped away in his car. A frantic chase ensued, which eventually resulted in Bruce running away from the police and into a river.

Several times, the police threw ropes to encourage Bruce to come out of the water. Each time, he would grab hold of it and pull himself a few metres back to shore but – realising that he would be detained – would return to the water again. Several police teams were joined by a couple of ambulance crews, ready to take him to the hospital. The helicopter was still hovering, illuminating the main character of this drama. Police divers were

---

[50] NHFD. National Hip Fracture Database 2021 [Available from: https://www.data.gov.uk/dataset/145cd65d-d109-4eab-8d20-ce0bd139f528/national-hip-fracture-database-annual-report-2021.

brought in to try to prevent Bruce from drowning when the inevitable loss of consciousness ensued.

After about an hour, Bruce's body gave up. Physically exhausted, he slumped into the water, and the divers prevented him from drowning. He was conscious but delirious and too tired to fight.

The paramedics assessed Bruce immediately. There were no obvious injuries, but his core temperature was under 30°C. He was severely hypothermic. Wet clothes were removed. A reflective blanket was put on. More cloth blankets were piled on. Within 30 minutes, he arrived in A&E. He was intubated and ventilated for a CT scan and then brought up to the ICU. Hot air blankets and warm intravenous fluids were used first. Then, warm bladder irrigation was commenced via a catheter. All the while, two police officers stood beside the bed, as is required for criminals requiring hospital treatment.

The next day, Bruce's temperature had risen to a normal level, and it was time to wake him up. To ensure the safety of staff and patient, his hands were handcuffed in a rigid figure of eight. Then, an alternative sedative agent was used to keep him calm while the main drugs were stopped. Four police officers stood at four corners of the bed. They turned their bodycams on. Three nurses started the process of waking Bruce up. It only took 15 minutes for him to begin to wake up.

His hands started moving first, but they were restricted by the handcuffs. Then his head started to turn from side to side. His eyes started flickering open and closed. He saw the police officers and felt the handcuffs and realised that he had been arrested. There was no point trying to escape. He was outnumbered and restrained. He was soon able to obey our commands and was ready to be extubated. Before long, Bruce began to boast, much to the disgust of all the staff present.

"Yeah, that f*king bitch. I took 'er by the f*king hair and dragged her outta the house!" he gloated. "Didn't care she was naked, just dragged her out the f*king house."

He taunted the police officers, hurled racist remarks at me, and slandered his girlfriend. Behind closed doors in the coffee room, the moral turmoil of having to treat an unrepentant criminal manifested in colourful exchanges among the nurses and doctors.

"What a scrote-bag," said a colleague, a slang for comparing Bruce to a scrotum.

"I wanted to just pull his catheter out with the balloon still inflated," remarked a nurse. This would have caused tremendous pain in his penis.

A fellow doctor joked that he wanted to inject Bruce with a paralysing agent and watch as he slowly suffocated and died. None of these things occurred. Instead, we demonstrated grace. Despite his history and circumstances, we cared for Bruce like any other patient. For a most undeserving candidate, large resources were utilised only for him to be put behind bars right after his discharge from hospital. From the police officers to the doctors, from the helicopters to the ventilators, from the physical destruction of vehicles to the verbal abuse of the staff. Perhaps society would be better off without Bruce, but I suspect even this outcome would not have been entirely satisfactory.

This struggle to show compassion and care to undeserving patients occurs more frequently than most people think. Many A&E colleagues complain about their departments filled with the drunk and the drugged, especially on weekends. Some of these patients require the immediate attention of several staff members for a considerable period, usually due to concerns about their consciousness levels. CT scans are often performed to rule out other causes of their stupor. This may involve several staff and usually takes about an hour. The radiologists would have to report the scans, and other health professionals may be involved, too.

Other patients swing to the opposite end of the spectrum and come into hospital kicking, swearing, punching, spitting and vomiting. They pose a different problem but are just as resource-intensive. Often, security staff are required to provide a deterrent to violence. Sometimes, such patients launch assaults on staff who are assessing them. Many colleagues have sustained broken spectacles, black eyes, bruised breasts or scratched arms from such encounters. Other times, patients use their bodily secretions and excretions as threats against the approach of healthcare staff. I have dealt with patients who were such a danger to themselves and staff that up to five security guards had to restrain them for me to use medications to sedate them and manage their care. There are those in between who are not violent, nor semi-comatose, but from whom getting a coherent story is frustrating, time-consuming, confusing, and sometimes impossible. These patients may attempt to tell a story and answer questions, but may take a long time to do so, or may be so inebriated that the brain is incapable of stringing words together to form sentences. The doctor may conclude that the patient is likely intoxicated but would be unable to rule out any serious issues within the skull, so may be forced to send the patient through a CT scanner, too. More radiation, more staff involved, more resources.

A subset of these patients will end up on the ICU. Usually, it is because they are so unconscious they are unable to maintain their own airway. They get intubated and ventilated for a day or so, until their bodies metabolise the toxins in their blood. At about £1,500 per patient per night, it really is an expensive night out.

I often think about the global inequalities of health. I remember Grace in Papua New Guinea and consider how, if she had received care similar to that of the little boy in the UK, she might have survived. She would be a teenager by now, maybe dreaming of changing the world, or making her parents proud in a dance show, or competing in a sport for the region or country even.

I think back to Mercy, who also probably would have survived and lived a long and productive life if she had received the same attention, investigations, and interventions that Pamela did in the UK.

I compare the resources used on Bruce and other inebriated patients with the sutures that Nathaniel's family had to buy in the middle of the night just to receive life-saving treatment for circumstances that were out of his control.

Then I start to remember the criminals I have treated and the drug addicts whose lives I have supported on ICU. Like many other frontline staff, I find it easy to complain about how time and resources are apparently being wasted on what many judge as undeserving patients. Sometimes, it is through gritted teeth that I perform my well-rehearsed show of compassion. I, too, have been brash to intoxicated patients. I have scolded and shouted at some for their unacceptable behaviour. I've secretly sniggered to myself when these patients get escorted by police officers into custody. Faced with resource pressures and heavy workloads, the grace which we are required to show to all patients sometimes seems more than what we can ever muster.

———◆◆◆———

When I reflect on my experiences in Papua New Guinea, Uganda, and several Southeast Asian countries, it is easy to understand why I continue to believe in and be thankful for the universal healthcare we have in the UK (and in many other high-income countries). But when it comes to the seemingly undeserving patient, I find that I need a conviction far deeper than Bevan's emotive words, and far more profound than the academic argument of "health for all". For me, it comes from a long history of similar commitment. In the 4th century, St Basil founded the Basiliad just outside of Caesarea to care for those ostracised by the Roman society: lepers, the elderly, the sick. His challenge then seems equally applicable today:

The bread which you hold back belongs to the hungry; the coat, which you guard in your locked storage chests, belongs to the naked; …The silver that you keep hidden in a safe place belongs to the one in need.[51]

Similarly, Islamic institutions during the Middle Ages specifically welcomed patients regardless of race, age, or economic status. Not to forget Mother Teresa's work in Calcutta in the late 1900s, the monastic hospitals in the UK which preceded the NHS, and the conviction of Henry Dunant, who founded and shaped the International Red Cross.[52,53] It is faith that compels me to care for the undeserving and underprivileged. Faith, and the example of brave men and women of faith. And, for me, the words and actions of the centre of my faith, *"Heal the*

---

[51] Heyne T. Reconstructing the world's first hospital: The Basiliad. Hektoen International. 2015;Spring.

[52] Aitken JT, Aitken JT, Fuller HWC, Johnson D, Christian Medical F. The Influence of Christians in medicine1984.

[53] Tan MZY. There is power in the blood. Hektoen International. 2020(Winter).

sick, raise the dead, cleanse those who have leprosy, drive out demons. Freely you have received; freely give." - Matthew 10:8

Therefore, despite the racist remarks hurled at me by Bruce. Despite being spat on by agitated patients or being punched and kicked by confused ones. Despite treating some patients repeatedly for self-inflicted problems, I will continue to hold the hand of yet another relapsing alcoholic, to lend an ear to the nth patient living in dire circumstances, and to care for many tricked and trapped by addiction. I will continue to love, to bless, to do good and to pray, because of the grace I have received myself.

> *"Amazing grace how sweet the sound that saved a wretch like me."*
> *- John Newton, 1779*

20. Silence is Not Golden

"Silence is golden" - English idiom

Silence is not golden. It does not shimmer, does not shine, is not precious. Silence in medicine is the loss of the normal sounds of bodily functions. It is the lack of the familiar rhythmic lub-dub of the heart valves, the stillness of no breath sounds, the blank canvas of the loss of capacity for consciousness. The silence which descends upon the medical team after a failed resuscitation attempt may be cold, may be heavy, may indeed be costly. But it certainly is not golden. Silence is the lack of life. Silence is death.

Even the temporary silence of skipped heartbeats, as in an arrhythmia, is disconcerting. As is the treatment for some arrhythmias like supraventricular tachycardias (SVT). In this condition, the heart may race up to 250 beats a minute, four times the normal heart rate. Patients feel severe palpitations and sometimes chest pain.

Before giving adenosine to treat the SVT, I tell patients they may feel like they are about to die. Adenosine resets the heart, and for a few seconds, their heart stops, the beeping of the monitor goes silent, everyone holds their breath in anticipation, watches the flat line on the monitor, feels the butterflies in their own stomachs, prays, waits a few more seconds – far too long for comfort – begins to feel like something should be done… and then the heart restarts. Those few seconds of cardiac standstill are agony for patients, whose eyes slowly grow wider and wider as they realise the suffocating silence. But this is a temporary state, mere seconds compared to the lasting silence of asystole, the flatline on the ECG, the cessation of cardiac activity, the loss of electrical conduction within the nerves and muscles of the heart. Death.

In the lungs, silence is the harbinger of death in life-threatening asthma and airway obstruction. First, the normal, quiet breath sounds are replaced with the wheeze of turbulence. Then, as the airways continue to spasm and constrict, less and less airflow is permitted. Finally, the dreaded "silent chest" ensues, all while imaginary deafening alarm bells ring in my head.

There is a helplessness in a patient's eyes when this occurs. Physiologically, their sympathetic tone increases, the so-called "fight or flight" response. Pupils dilate, heart rate increases, and blood pressure rises; their bodies perceive the threat to life. Emotionally, it is the classic *angor animi* (anguish of the soul): the perception of dying. Mentally, it is the acute silence of suspense, the looking over a cliff just before a fatal drop. This silence is unnerving. The Norwegian artist Edvard Munch perhaps best captures it in his iconic painting *The Scream*. Viewed in the hushed surroundings of the National Gallery, this still painting portrays the horror on the faces of such patients. But maybe the wavy, crimson skies best represent the intense cerebral turbulence. After all, the small inscription of *"perhaps this is painted by a madman"* on the clouds in the painting equally reflects the irrational behaviour of a hypoxic patient.

Once the mind is starved of oxygen, panic ensues. Patients attempt to scream, but without sufficient airflow, no noise is emitted. They grab at anything, clutch at straws, hang on for dear life. I know the emergency about to occur and prepare for the worst. Emergency drugs, tubes of various sizes, additional airway equipment, anaesthetic agents, muscle relaxants, infusion pumps… and machines; only the hum of a ventilator stills the silent scream.

Deadly silence is not confined to the heart or lungs. Even for the seemingly less "vital" organ, the bowels, silence can be just as pathological. We think of bowel sounds as inconveniences. Society expects us to be embarrassed by the rasp of flatulence, excuse ourselves for the gurgling of hunger, or suppress the rumble of a burp. But the general surgeons will confess that they celebrate the fart. The release of flatulence provides reassurance that the bowels are working.

For the patient with severe abdominal pain and a diagnosis of bowel obstruction, flatulence means that the bowels are not completely blocked nor perforated. It usually means the patient is not critically ill, nor is major emergency surgery likely needed. For the post-operative patient who has had part of their bowels resected, flatulence indicates the resumption of normal bowel passage. The gurgling of the bowels foretells the beginnings of movement and passage: small inklings of recovery.

On the contrary, the absence of bowel sounds in post-operative patients may indicate ileus. In ileus, the bowels go on strike, protesting a surgeon's unwelcome handling or groping by refusing to carry out its normal peristaltic function.[54] Without peristalsis, food and drink remain in the stomach and cause bloating, nausea and vomiting. There is poor absorption, leading to malnutrition. The growth of abnormal bacteria and a build-up of gas may then lead to further bowel dilation.

In severe cases, the dilated bowels exert upward pressure on the diaphragm, leading to shortness of breath and difficulty breathing. I have taken care of many patients with ileus. They can spend weeks on the ICU due to nutritional problems, electrolyte imbalances and infectious complications. So, rejoice in flatulence. Hallelujah for borborygmi (the medical term for bowel gurgling). Sing and be glad for eructation (also known as the belch). For the mutterings of the guts are songs of joy when compared with the silent problems that ileus brew.

Silence is not golden. Then again, there is sometimes a calm about silence, the fading into nothingness, the last whispers of life which usher in the afterlife.

Death: the irreversible loss of capacity of consciousness and the loss of capacity for breathing. - Academy of Medical Royal Colleges, 2008.

I memorised this definition for my anaesthetic exams. It was neat, clinical, sterile – simple words for a simple phenomenon. Indeed, the first few deaths I witnessed were calm and silent. My first job as a brand-new foundation doctor was on a geriatric ward. Unsurprisingly, several patients had come to the end of their lives and died during their hospital stays.

Their deaths were all expected. Do-Not-Attempt-Cardio-Pulmonary-Resuscitation (DNACPR) orders were signed early, and they were allowed to die. Instead of the back-to-back bleeps, the countless phone calls, and the tens of thousands of steps taken running from ward to ward for mundane jobs, verifying a death was a morbidly welcome break from the chaos of being

---

[54] Peristalsis refers to the normal, rhythmic contractions of the gut which propel food and drink forward, from the oesophagus all the way to the rectum. Gurgling of the bowels are sounds produced by normal peristalsis.

the ward on-call foundation doctor at night. It was a quiet alternative to otherwise messy resuscitation attempts. So, I dutifully took the patient notes, put on my apron and gloves, and solemnly let myself in the room. Sometimes, I would even knock on the door, out of habit, but then I realised how silly that must have seemed to anyone else. Silence, while not particularly golden, was at least appreciated, even if only by the junior doctor.

The rituals surrounding the verification of these deaths were strange. Inside the room or cubicle of a recently deceased patient is silence. The curtains are always drawn, and it is frequently dim. By the time I got there, the nurses would usually have made sure that the patient was neatly tucked into bed. The blanket was always immaculately folded at the chest or sometimes the waist. The arms were sometimes tucked under the sheets or sometimes laid above them. Their hair was frequently nicely combed.

The room was always spotless. Monitors turned off, tray-table squared off to the bed or in a corner, personal artefacts, if present, always laid out beautifully. There was an intrinsic order to the conduct and presentation of death, and the nurses always performed fantastically. I would approach the corpse in quiet reverence, just as the body had been treated by the nurses prior to my arrival. I would then speak the patient's name while squeezing their shoulder. This confirms their unresponsiveness. I proceeded to gently open their eyelids and shine a bright torch in them. This tests the reflex arcs of the eyes. Following this, I then put my fingers on the neck and my stethoscope on the chest. I would then observe three minutes of silence – three minutes of ensuring there were no breath sounds, no carotid pulse, and no heart sounds. After this, I had a habit of whispering "rest in peace" before I left the room. I would then write in the notes:

No heart sounds
No breath sounds
No carotid pulse
For 3 minutes.
Pupils fixed and dilated.
Death verified at [time]

Maybe this silence was precious. It helped me focus on the patient before me, ensuring that I did not miss a heartbeat or a final breath (there were never missed heartbeats or breaths). It took me away from my clinical duties in a short, precious final encounter with one who had ceased to be. It provided time for ritual, tradition, and reflection.

These experiences were serene and calm, just as how many near-death experiences have been recalled, according to psychiatrist Bruce Greyson's book *After.*[55] His research demonstrated that numerous patients who have recovered from cardiac arrests, and thus near-death experiences, describe feelings of warmth and comfort. This is completely opposite from an actual scene of a cardiac arrest. Oftentimes, there is panic, dread and chaos amongst the medical team. Shouts and firm commands are common. Medical packaging is usually littered all around the bed and floor. Intubation is sometimes performed without anaesthetic drugs (because the patient is indeed already completely unconscious). CPR looks barbaric. Multiple professionals are usually involved in a tight environment, squeezing past each other, performing various tasks. There is little concern for aesthetics or civility during a cardiac arrest.

Yet, according to Greyson, patients are frequently unaware of the chaos. Instead, they may describe muted sounds or silence, outer-body experiences, or the warmth and comfort of a cocoon. They may see light or hear their name softly called. In other words, the patient's experience of near-death, and perhaps by extension, death, may not mirror the healthcare professionals' experiences. However, our conduct surrounding death is of such vital importance that the cultural insensitivities demonstrated by international teams during the Ebola epidemic of 2014 were cited as a key factor for unanticipated healthcare avoidance

---

[55] Greyson B. After: a doctor explores what near-death experiences reveal about life and beyond: Penguin; 2021.

behaviour and, therefore, increased spread of the disease.[56] The ripples of death thus spread far wider than just the deceased.

During my intensive care medicine training, I learnt that death is sometimes not quite as packaged as those I had verified on my geriatric placement. It still contained all the information in the statement, but it was not simply a few lines of illegible scrawl in a patient's notes, nor was it completely silent. Five years after graduating from medical school, I was involved in diagnosing brainstem death in one of my patients.

Brainstem death occurs when the part of the brain which controls automatic functions is irreversibly damaged. Often, this happens because of severe traumatic head injury, but it sometimes also occurs with hypoxic brain injury, where the brain has a period of lack of blood flow or oxygen. This may be the case with a cardiac arrest, respiratory depression, or prolonged neurological disorder. There is frequently little damage to the other vital organs. This means the heart continues to beat. Breathing and oxygenation are almost always maintained by a ventilator on ICU. However, there is no prospect of recovery. The definition of death includes those who are brainstem dead, but the diagnosis is done in a different way: by testing the automatic responses or reflexes of the cranial nerves, as well as the function of the respiratory centre in the brainstem.

Fran was a 70-year-old lady who was brought into hospital after suffering a collapse and cardiac arrest. The paramedics achieved the return of spontaneous circulation after some CPR, and she was then intubated in A&E. When she had a CT head scan, it revealed a severe subarachnoid haemorrhage (a spontaneous bleed into her brain). This sudden event dramatically increased the sympathetic response (fight or flight),

---

[56] Southall et al.'s paper analysed the international aid responses during the Ebola outbreak in Liberia in 2014. Locals soon realised infected persons would be forcibly isolated in insufficiently-staffed and poorly-resourced emergency treatment centres, often with poor communication channels with their families. This contrasts with the family support they were used to providing in their local hospitals (see the chapter *Grace*). The result was mistrust between the locals and the international teams, hiding of family members, and worsening of the spread of Ebola. Southall HG, DeYoung SE, Harris CA. Lack of Cultural Competency in International Aid Responses: The Ebola Outbreak in Liberia. Front Public Health. 2017;5:5.

and due to the physiological stress, her heart stopped. But even though her heart was restarted by CPR, by the time she got to A&E, she was showing signs of brainstem death. The subarachnoid haemorrhage was so severe that the additional blood in the skull forced the brainstem downward through the little hole where it normally exits the skull. This increase in pressure subsequently caused irreversible damage to the brainstem nerves. Luckily, the bleeding did not continue and although she did not improve, neither did she deteriorate. After three days of making sure there was no significant recovery potential, we proceeded to perform brainstem death testing. As the ICU registrar on the unit, I was asked to be the second physician performing the test with my consultant (this is a legal requirement). It was also a key skill developed during intensive care training.

My consultant quizzed me on all the reflexes tested. We then prepared all the equipment and the brainstem death testing protocol for reference. We made sure all her respiratory and metabolic parameters were normalised prior to the test. This ensures nothing else can contribute to the lack of consciousness. Finally, the tests were carried out.

Pupillary reflex: A bright light was shone in each eye, testing the optic nerve and the oculomotor nerve. Her pupils were fixed and dilated.

Corneal reflex: A small piece of cotton wool was brushed against her eye, testing the trigeminal and facial nerves. She did not blink.

Pain response: Pressure is applied to the supraorbital ridge (eyebrow ridge), testing again the trigeminal and facial nerves. There was no response.

Caloric reflex: Ice-cold water is flushed into the ear, testing the vestibulocochlear and the abducens nerves. Normally, this will activate the former, causing an involuntary deviation of the eyes towards the side of the flushing. Her eyes remained fixed in a neutral position.

Pharyngeal or gag reflex: The back of the throat is stimulated, testing the trigeminal or glossopharyngeal nerve, and the vagus nerve. There was no gag.

Cough reflex: The trachea is stimulated with a suction catheter from the endotracheal tube, testing the vagus nerve. There was no cough.

Throughout these tests, the ventilator continued to control Fran's breathing. I could hear the soft hum of the turbines during each respiratory cycle. The monitoring told us that her oxygen saturations were still 100%, and her respiratory rate was set at 12 breaths per minute. Along with it, her heart continued to beat. I saw her chest move ever so slightly with each beat. I saw the trace of the arterial line on the monitor correspond to each beat of her heart. There was no real silence. I remember thinking to myself,

"There are still signs of life! She's not dead!" and I was right. She wasn't dead. Not yet.

We proceeded to perform the last test, the *Apnoea test.* This tests the respiratory centres, the automatic parts of the brain which control breathing. We took a blood gas to ensure that parameters were within range. Then, we provided some supplemental oxygen, stopped the ventilator and disconnected the breathing circuit from the endotracheal tube. We then stood in silence, watching for any chest movement. There was none. But it wasn't silent. Her heart continued to beat; the barely audible "lub-dub" betrayed the silence of death I was used to previously. The carbon dioxide in her blood slowly rose to a prerequisite level.

Then the test was over.

There were no breath efforts. Fran was connected back to the ventilator, to the familiar hum. Parameters: normal. Yet, she was now legally dead. We then went into the relatives' room, where Fran's son Chris was waiting. The news was broken. There were tears of loss but not of shock. He had been prepared for this. We had spoken to him several times over the previous three days. The organ donation specialist nurse was also involved and had explained the donation process. Fran was to be an organ donor. Her heart, lungs and kidneys would be procured for donation. We then ushered Chris in with us, who wanted to be present when we performed the second set of confirmatory brainstem death tests.

That evening, after Chris and the rest of the family had said their last goodbyes, Fran went to theatre for organ donation. The transplant team had arrived from several different hospitals to procure Fran's heart, lungs and kidneys. The hubbub of activity caused by the huge team seemed almost irreverent to the situation.

The logistics of organ donation and transplant are exceedingly complex. Organ donation specialist nurses must investigate the suitability of organs prior to theatre. They then communicate with several centres that may (or may not) accept the organ. This has to be done and confirmed at several points during the procurement process. They ensure all lines of communication are maintained, and protocols for transfer are adhered to, aiming to preserve the procured organ in the best condition possible.

With Fran, two cardiothoracic surgeons managed the heart and lungs with their own scrub nurse. Two other general transplant surgeons dealt with the kidneys with their own scrub nurse, too. My anaesthetic consultant and I maintained organ physiology and anaesthesia. Several other members of the theatre team ensured supplies and equipment were available. The theatre, which normally felt spacious, suddenly seemed claustrophobic with the myriad of equipment and personnel from the various specialties. We had all been briefed prior to theatre. Plans were confirmed again, and the last checks made. Then, the procurement began.

Throughout the procurement surgery, there was a baseline buzz of activity and noise. Careful dissection was performed on the organs. We, as the anaesthetists, continued to titrate the various infusions to maintain blood pressure. We monitored all the vital parameters and adjusted the ventilator settings. The heart and lungs were exposed and freed from all the surrounding tissue in preparation for clamping and removal. Then, the cardiothoracic surgeons took a break to wait for the general surgeons to fully expose and prepare the kidneys. Once everything was ready, they re-scrubbed and donned their sterile attire. The lungs were clamped at their origins as we turned off the ventilator. No more breath sounds. No more ventilator hum. Silence. Not quite. The aorta was clamped. Heart beating. Beating. Slowing down. Fibrillating. Stopping. Stopped. Silence.

The voices of multiple surgeons seemed disproportionately loud against the silence of the body.

This was no silence of death.

The cessation of life for Fran was soon to be the beginning of new life for several recipients of her organs. Over the next hour, her organs were dissected, examined, confirmed and placed into specialised containers for transport. Already, the multiple recipients had been informed and made their way into various hospitals around the country in preparation for the implantation of the donor organs. The end of Fran's chapter was the start of several new chapters. Three months later, we received a letter from the organ donation team explaining that Fran's organs had been successfully donated to several patients, who were all doing very well.

After the organ procurement, I sat down in the staff room and sipped my tea. In the silence, I considered the new lease of life for those recipients of Fran's organs. And I thought to myself,

"*This* silence... is golden."

"Their beginning was their end, and their end was their beginning."
- TS Eliot's East Coker.

21. Painting an ICU

"[Monet was] only an eye - yet what an eye" - Paul Cézanne

The on-call room in North Manchester General Hospital was utilitarian. Like many other on-call rooms, it had a simple bed, a shower, and a toilet. It overlooked the public car park, and while this meant I could hear all the cars passing the hospital, at least I had somewhere to lie down, which was more than what I had in some other hospitals. A single picture frame hung above the bed. It was a print of Monet's water lilies. Perhaps one of his most famous sets of work, the water lilies series, not only provides a timeline for the manifestations of Monet's worsening cataracts but also chronicles the evolution of the artistic genre accredited to him: impressionism.

Much has been written about Monet's ophthalmic pathology.[57,58,59,60] His diary chronicled the deterioration of his eyesight due to cataracts and his fear of potentially losing his sight altogether with surgery. The delay in surgery, coupled with his love of painting the plants and flowers around the pond and Japanese bridge in his garden, provided a detailed and longitudinal glimpse into the effects of cataracts.

The first paintings of the series, completed in 1898, detail the hues of pink and yellow toward the centre of the lilies. Each flower stands out from the dark background of the water. The lily pads are painted blue and green, and their edges softly blend into the water they so effortlessly float above. In some paintings, these same edges are highlighted in arcs of orange and yellow, reflections from the rising or setting sun. In other paintings, the water contains the shimmering purple-red reflections of the so-called "magic hour" lighting at dusk.

By 1903, several paintings demonstrated the cloudiness of vision from the initial stages of cataracts. This cloudiness is

---

[57] Hajar R. Monet and Cataracts. Heart Views. 2016;17(1):40-1.

[58] Gruener A. The effect of cataracts and cataract surgery on Claude Monet. Br J Gen Pract. 2015;65(634):254-5.

[59] Kopplin P. Monet and his cataracts. Hektoen International. 2016;9(1).

[60] Metzler S. Monet's illnesses: beyond cataracts. Hektoen International. 2020;13(1).

concentrated toward the centre of the paintings, manifesting as softer edges, more prominent whites within the reflections in the water, and a translucency akin to viewing through a sheer screen. Between 1906 and 1915, the paintings continue to evolve, taking on increasingly redder tints and sepia tones. This corresponds with maturing cataracts, which reduce the ability to see blues and greens, and accentuate browns and reds. It is particularly prominent in the railings of the Japanese bridge, which were green but often painted brown or red in the paintings of 1920-1922, prior to his cataract surgery.

Two paintings, currently displayed in New York and Houston, epitomise the late stages of Monet's cataracts. The predominant palette consisted of dark browns, oranges, yellows, and reds. The bridge railings are wavy, bold, and almost black. The willow no longer sways, and the plants seem to blend into a mini jungle at the edges of the pond. Brushstrokes are broad, distinct, and jarring. The turmoil and frustration boil over and make the painting feel like a fiery furnace rather than a soothing scene.

In 1874, at least 15 years before his Water Lilies series (which forms the backdrop to his medical diagnosis), his famous painting *Impression, Sunrise* drew scathing criticism from art critic Louis Leroy, who described it as a partially finished wallpaper and – in essence – unwittingly coined the Impressionist movement.[61]

Contrary to Leroy's criticisms, Monet purposefully diverged from the then widely accepted practice of idealising a scene when painting. He considered light and its effect on colours and movement and its effect on visual perception. He began painting outdoor scenes and would paint with wet paint over wet paint, dramatically widening the range of contrasts, textures, and depths he could achieve. Central to the Impressionist philosophy was the artist's own perception of the scene, which included the

[61] Prodger M. The man who made Monet: how impressionism was saved from obscurity London: The Guardian; 2015 [Available from: https://www.theguardian.com/artanddesign/2015/feb/21/the-man-who-made-monet-how-impressionism-was-saved-from-obscurity.

influence of environmental conditions, lighting, and his/her own emotions.[62,63]

Impressionism predated Monet's cataracts and continued after his cataract surgery in 1922. His perception of colours and outlines improved dramatically, but his paintings continued to lean into the impressionism he was so famous for. Despite the return of blues and greens, his paintings were built upon countless minute brushstrokes, forming overarching masterpieces far exceeding the sum of its parts. This was the genius of Monet, and this progression – from exquisite detail to one of "meta-complexity" – seemed to also parallel my own training in intensive care medicine and that of the journeys of some of my patients.

━━━◆◆━━━

In medical school, I was obsessed with details. Wanting to know everything, I pored over textbooks, looking for the next nugget of knowledge. Fascinated by the intricacies of the human body, I looked up each syndrome, learned each blood test I came across, and memorised the finer details of anatomy. From Aspergers and Alport syndromes to Z-lines and ZAP70, the study of medicine seemed clear cut. A particular constellation of symptoms and signs may be associated with a certain disease caused by a single genetic mutation. Understanding some of the body's biochemical pathways allows us to target specific drugs. It was logical, linear, and lucid. If only one knew all the labels, pathways and interactions, medicine could be mastered.

This reductionistic approach to the study of medicine was both empowering and suppressive. Breaking down the unfathomable complexity of the human body into fundamental constituents seems to empower mere mortals to push the frontiers of scientific understanding. Linnaeus' taxonomical hierarchy provided a structure with which to distinguish morphological differences between species, genus, and family. Watson and Crick's discovery of the building blocks of DNA has formed the basis for the entire field of genetic medicine.

---

[62] Goetz A, Sander E. Monet at Giverny: Gourcuff Gradenigo; 2015.

[63] Tate. Impressionism New York: Tate Gallery; 2021 [Available from: https://www.tate.org.uk/art/art-terms/i/impressionism.

Within medical training, the stepwise consideration of organ systems continues to be a predictor of success in our numerous postgraduate examinations. When answering questions about disease processes, successful candidates almost unanimously processed and presented their thoughts using an organ systems approach. For example, the implications of anaesthetising an infant can be explained through the differences in their airways, cardiovascular, respiratory, gastrointestinal, renal, central nervous systems, and so on.

Yet, at times, this seemingly universal philosophy within science fails to consider the entirety of human experience. The complexity of human pathology, the irrationality of human behaviour, and the unpredictability of critical illness defy the rigid attempts of reductionism to classify and categorise. Medicine, if practised with a purely reductionist approach, would indeed be suppressive, going against the Hippocratic oath to "do no harm or *injustice*."

As I progressed through general and then specialty training, I began to learn more about the intricacies of medicine and the inadequacy of the reductionist thought process. The spreadsheet of blood tests displayed on the computer during a ward round may provide quantitative biomarker information on each individual organ, but it does not provide a sufficient assessment about the state of a patient. Instead of trying to correct every test result to normality, I found my perception changing. I started looking at patients and their quality of life, instead of only whether they would live or die.

I explored their priorities, their social networks, and their spiritual needs. Taking these into account allowed me to build a fuller, richer, and more holistic clinical picture, one that would enable me to make better and more humane decisions. This was the art of medicine. The history was my scene, the examination my brushes and investigations were my paints. I became an impressionist.

A few years ago, I also learned that this progression was not confined to the artist or the physician. Instead, I was seeing the development of impressionism in my patient's loved one…

———◆◆———

Gurjit was a frail, elderly gentleman who had several co-morbidities limiting his daily function. When he developed severe pneumonia, he was intubated and ventilated in the ICU. One by one, his organs started to fail. We were pessimistic about his prognosis, so I spoke to his son Billal on the phone to voice my concerns about his father's critical condition.

"Your father is needing a lot of oxygen on the ventilator. He is also needing medications to keep his blood pressure up." I explained.

"What are his saturations?" Billal asked.

"94%, but he is needing high levels of oxygen to keep it at that level. Do you work in healthcare?" I asked.

"I'm a pharmacist. I live in Germany, but I'm also the only family Dad has."

"Well, he is critically ill from a severe chest infection. As such, he has a significant chance of dying. But, at the moment, his other organs seem to be holding up."

"Oh, what is his CRP and white cell count then?"

"They were fairly high, but we shall see if the antibiotics help."

Billal wanted to know the exact blood results and observations. After the conversation, I couldn't help feeling that Billal had failed to grasp the gravity of his father's predicament. A few days later, Gurjit failed to make any clinical progress. He was still ventilated, but he needed more vasopressors to maintain his blood pressure. Again, I spoke to Billal to try to explain the deterioration.

"But his saturations are now 95%. His CRP and white cell count are coming down. How can he be deteriorating?" came an unbelieving voice across the phone.

It seemed Billal was unable to comprehend the fact that his father was not making clinical progress. Mildly frustrated at his lack of understanding, I persevered by explaining that although his saturations were better, he was needing more oxygen. While the inflammatory markers were marginally better, other organs were beginning to show signs of deterioration.

Within a couple of days, Gurjit's kidneys failed. His urine output gradually declined. His blood tests suggested that his liver was slowly failing, also demonstrated externally by the yellowish tinge in the whites of his eyes. He continued to require heavy support for both his lungs and heart. This was going to be a terminal event. It was unanimously decided that Gurjit was dying and that our priorities needed to shift toward palliation. So, I called Billal again.

Again, the telephone conversation began with several questions about blood results and observations. Without visual and environmental input from a physical visit to the ICU, Billal struggled to picture his critically ill father.[64] He failed to appreciate the number of lines and medications needed to maintain his blood pressure. He was unable to see the change in skin colour of his father – one of the tell-tale signs of a deteriorating patient. Over the telephone, the overwhelming sensory experience of a visit to ICU seemed diminished, dampened, and dulled.

Several iterations later, it finally dawned on Billal that his father was indeed dying. The most sophisticated technologies were unable to save him. Then, the questions began to change. Instead of the minute detail, Billal was able to form an impression of the situation. Through the course of the conversation, Billal began to abandon his questions about minute details of blood results and observations. In a Monet-like fashion, he started to develop an overall impression of his dying father, building up his mental image of illness, sickness and death. In a similar fashion, I guided Billal to integrate and assimilate the clinical data we had collected on Gurjit over the last few days, encouraging him to form an overall impression of his deteriorating father, just as we had done amongst the clinical team.

"How will he die? How long does he have? Will he be in pain?"

"It's impossible to determine how long he will live, but four of his main organs are failing. We need to think about changing priorities to make him comfortable. We have medications which can help with pain and other symptoms associated with the dying process. He will not be suffering."

"I will fly in tomorrow to see him, but I'm not sure what to expect. I've never been to an ICU before."

---

[64] See the COVID-19 supplement towards the end of this book.

I painted a picture of an ICU over the phone, an overall impression à la Monet. Broad strokes of the environment, from the machines to the monitors. I filled in the muted colours – lines that were inserted into Billal's father. Then, the lights and shadows – the various beeps and alarms he might see and hear, the decisions to be made and the journey to death. I told Billal that a staff member would be with him, guiding him, much as I had prepared him for his visit.

The next day, as Billal stood in front of his dying father, his mind painted one last scene. Gone was the focus on vital signs. No longer were the intricacies of blood results important. Just like Monet, Billal's impression of his father was now filled with a more irregular palette, darker hues, blurred lines, and patchy reflections. The fatherly constant in Billal's life was now merely a fleeting frame of a bridge. Comfortable, assuaged, and with his loved one beside him, I was now confident that Gurjit would die with dignity. This, I hoped, would form a beautiful final impression.

"Like a bridge over troubled waters,
I will lay me down…"
- Simon and Garfunkel

[An extract of this was an honourable mention in the Hektoen International Grand Prix 2021. Tan MZY. Painting an ICU. Hektoen International. 2021;13. Available from: [https://hekint.org/2021/08/19/painting-an-icu/] Used with permission.]

22. Beyond Bach

Polyrhythm

"We don't talk about such things!" - Daddy Tan

This was the conversation killer. The shatterer of opportunities. The silencer of desires. With this phrase, I didn't raise the subject again. It was not until several years later that I revisited the topic while writing a few articles.

The setting was Singapore. The person was my grandmother. I called her Mámà (嫲嫲). The first is a rising tone, and the second is a falling one. The score was death and dying. The underlying rhythm was an uncomfortable one. In this case, it was complete heart block. 嫲嫲 was recently diagnosed.

She had an episode of fainting, and when the doctors did an electrocardiogram (ECG), or heart tracing, it demonstrated a disconnect between the rhythm of the four chambers of the heart. Her ventricles only pumped at 30 beats a minute, while her atria pumped at 100 beats a minute. The resultant polyrhythm was irregular and unpredictable. The atria and ventricles sometimes beat together, counteracting each other. This meant little blood was ejected from the heart to the lungs or the rest of the body. It caused the heart to swell and the blood to swirl in chaotic streams of turbulence.

Listening to the heart of someone with heart block resembles a polyrhythmic piece of music. There is tension between musicians playing different rhythms, seemingly out-of-sync. A soundscape that makes you uncomfortable even though it is difficult to really put your finger on why. It reminds me of a visit to the House of Terror in Budapest, Hungary. The museum contained exhibits related to the fascist and communist regimes in Hungarian history. It takes an almost haunted house approach to the topic through a variety of techniques designed to make the visitor feel as if they were experiencing a nightmare. In one room, there was a Soviet-issue car on a rotating pedestal. The exhibition notes described the abduction of victims by secret police officers. A translucent dark curtain partially obscured the car, while a spotlight intermittently illuminated the seat. But it was really the music, composed by Ákos Kovács, that set my then-girlfriend into a state of unease to the point that she promptly exited without even reading the descriptions. The overhead speakers on the ceiling played a heavily distorted, grungy, and unrelenting piece of music. The guitar, bass and drums entered an everlasting loop. The seemingly regular 4 | 4 rhythm lured her into a false sense of familiarity. But then, after every alternate bar, the pattern repeated slightly earlier than expected. It was a 7 | 8 bar of music. This completely threw off the pattern her brain latched onto. It made her nauseous, and within three loops, she had to leave.

嫲嫲's heart block meant that even though both her atria and ventricles pumped at roughly predictable rhythms, they were not in sync, causing missed beats, extra sounds, and strange murmurs. She was prone to fainting episodes and at higher risk of sudden death. But she refused the pacemaker offered that would resynchronise the heart, "I'm old. I've had a good life. I am ready to go and be with 公公 (gong gong)," she said in Hokkien dialect, referring to her late husband, my grandfather, who died several years before.

嫲嫲 was 90 years old then. She was no longer the active woman she once was. Her severe scoliosis meant that her spine was so curved that she walked with an obvious limp. This had stopped her teaching tai chi a few years prior. She used to do this every morning, to many other residents in her block of flats. It was her way of staying active and maintaining community. Instead, she spent more time playing Tetris on her little Nintendo Game Boy. It so happened that my family and I were back in Singapore a few weeks after she was diagnosed with complete heart block. I noticed she wasn't looking as spritely as she used to during my previous visits home from the UK.

Knowing the prognosis of complete heart block and the likely progression of the condition, I felt compelled to discuss care preferences with 嫲嫲. Yet, I was unable to, not due to a loss of words but rather an inability to hold such nuanced discussions in a different language.

There is a strange linguistic phenomenon in the history of Singapore. My paternal grandparents were the second generation of migrants from China. 公公 and 嫲嫲 spoke the dialect Hokkien as a primary language. This was the main language spoken by their parents, who migrated from the Fujian province of China to Singapore. 公公 and 嬷嬷 also spoke Mandarin Chinese, but less fluently than Hokkien.

Both my parents were third-generation Singaporeans. During their childhood, in the 1960s to 70s, when Singapore was trying to build itself as the Antioch of the East, the government strongly encouraged its population to learn English. As a result, Mandarin Chinese and its various dialects were discouraged in favour of the Queen's English as a post-colonial nation. This was despite the history of British abandonment when the Japanese troops invaded Singapore during World War II, I might add. My father and mother, therefore, spoke firstly English, secondly Mandarin Chinese (although they could not write), and thirdly, Hokkien and Teochew (the dialect of my mother's ancestors).

When I was growing up, Singapore decided instead to promote multiculturalism and multi-racialism. The government, therefore, reversed their previous attempts and reintroduced mother tongues in school to encourage Singaporeans to speak different languages. So strong was their commitment that official documents and speeches had to be made in all four official languages: English, Mandarin Chinese, Malay, and Tamil. During secondary school, I – like all my classmates – could recite the Singapore pledge in all four languages. Our national anthem is in Malay. Our prime ministers have a long history of delivering their national day speeches in at least two languages. We have national public holidays that honour all four major religions in the country: Buddhism, Islam, Christianity, and Hinduism. But I never really learnt Hokkien, and I was never really good at Mandarin Chinese either.

Contrapuntal

I was confident in talking to patients about diagnoses, prognoses, medical technologies, death and dying in English. After all, I had about 15 years of medical training for that. I yearned to discuss these topics with 嬷嬷 so that her healthcare providers could deliver compassionate, realistic care that aligned with her values. But I could not do it in Mandarin Chinese, let alone Hokkien. Because of this language barrier, I had a somewhat distant relationship with my grandparents. Both sets of grandfathers could speak limited English, and that, in combination with my broken Mandarin Chinese, was only sufficient to make small talk. My grandmother did not speak English.

So, I did what I thought was the second-best option: I talked to my father and other relatives. I told them about complete heart block. I explained the prognosis and likely cause of death. I said that 嬤嬤 had a significant risk of her heart suddenly stopping. I then went on to describe, as best as I could, what would happen in that scenario. I recounted the numerous cardiac arrest situations I have been in. I told them, just like in the pages of this book, how ribs may be broken, tubes and lines may be inserted, and machines may be used, all for a very futile attempt to resuscitate a frail, 90-year-old woman who chose not to have a pacemaker in the first place. I then asserted, "I think you should talk to her about a do not attempt cardiopulmonary resuscitation (DNACPR) order."

"We don't talk about such things," was the blunt reply.

"But…" I went on to reiterate some of what I said.

"I know, but we just don't speak about it."

I was disappointed and scared. Disappointed that despite explanations about the trauma associated with resuscitation, I was unable to convince the family to discuss a DNACPR order. Scared that 嬤嬤 would end up in a futile resuscitation situation, and that the family may have to witness a traumatic and unnecessary intervention. To me, the situation seemed to epitomise this quote from Elif Shafak's novel *10 Minutes 38 Seconds in a Strange World*:

> *"How pathetic it was to try to relegate death to the periphery of life when death was at the centre of everything."*

I wanted 嬤嬤 to have what palliative care specialist Dr Kathryn Mannix described as a "normal" death in her book *With the End in Mind*. She writes about the tiredness and sleepiness. She explores the physiology behind the slowing and occasional cessation of breathing. She explains the normal process of fluctuating consciousness, and the frequently comfortable, gentle ways people exit life. Finally, she demonstrates the role of palliative care not only in symptomatic control towards the end of life but also in helping to empower patients and relatives to reclaim the relational processes around death. Mannix explains normal dying, so people fear it less.

These were not the deaths I knew. Biased by my professional experiences, coupled with my inability to discuss the issue directly, I feared that 嬷嬷 might be subject to painful, futile interventions out of her control. I felt that the silence assumed far too much, like one of the stories Mannix tells in her book about a lady who had terminal cancer. The patient's husband avoided talking about the topic out of love, and with the mistaken assumption that his wife was not aware of the severity of her own condition. On the other hand, she thought that he avoided the topic because he himself was unaware that her illness was terminal. They had reached an impasse when Kathryn was called. She spoke to each of them separately and then addressed both parties together. What followed was an epiphanic, tender moment of realisation that they both were actually thinking similar thoughts and grappling with similar fears. The ensuing conversations reignited the couple's commitment and intimacy with each other that had been fundamental to their several-decade-long marriage – vows that they continued to upkeep till death did them part.

We took several photos of 嬷嬷 during that trip to Singapore. My wife and I knew it would be the last time we saw her. I did not broach the topic of dying again during that trip. The linguistic barrier seemed compounded by a firm, deeply rooted cultural barrier. Then, when we returned to the UK, a third barrier – geographical separation – sealed my attempts. Isolated and sound-proofed, my dissonant cries fell out of harmony with the rest of the family's melody. Our rhythms did not groove, and our chords did not sound as one. To me, my family's avoidance of discussing death seemed divergent from 嬷嬷's mindset. She was the one who chose not to have a pacemaker. She said she wanted to be reunited with her husband. She knew that one day her life would come to an end, and with that wisdom, she did not attempt to avoid death but instead faced it and even dared to embrace it.

"I am ready to go and be with 公公 (gong gong)…"

Cadence

After we returned to the UK, the extended family, armed with the knowledge of 嫲嫲's likely progression, increased the frequency of their visits. They met up regularly in her little third-floor flat. They shared meals and fellowship. Conversations were aplenty, and the atmosphere was frequently bustling with the voices of uncles and aunties, nephews and nieces, and great-grandchildren. It was almost as if Chinese New Year had come around again, along with the reunion meals, the snacks, the photos, the incense, and the warmth of family life. When death approached, life swelled, concentrated, and mingled.

It reminded me of the last chapters and epilogue to Dr Paul Kalanithi's autobiography *When Breath Becomes Air*, which describes how, in the last months of his terminal illness, his extended family temporarily moved closer to spend time together. The feeling of warmth and the bonds of love characterised his terminal illness journey, particularly after the initial drugs failed. In the end, he took a courageous decision not to continue with intensive care or invasive therapies, and to focus on what is known as "best supportive care". For him, this meant taking off the oxygen and non-invasive ventilation, and switching instead to a morphine infusion to control breathlessness. In the presence of family, he slowly drifted away.

One day, I got a text from my mother,

"嫲嫲 died in her sleep. The paramedics came, but she was already dead. We are preparing for the funeral now."

Oh, the relief I felt! Yes, of course, there was sadness for the loss of my grandmother, but more overwhelmingly, a sense of relief that she had not been subject to futile CPR. Most of the extended family, even though sad, did not have prolonged grieving periods either. Those frequent visits had, in a way, prepared the family for 嫲嫲's death. Even though death was not discussed, it was very much present and central during those final months. It brought the family together and strengthened their relationships. It involved all parties, from young to old. It was familiar. Just as death ought to be.[65]

Re-examining myself, I then began to wonder if the extended family had been playing a beautiful symphony all along, and my attempts to force explicit discussions around DNACPR were, in fact, usurping the melody. Was I imposing my own cultural expectations onto 嫲嫲's care? Had I turned their music into my own concerto? Having spent my professional training life in the UK, I had become familiar with a culture of medicalising death. I had plenty of experiences where patients who probably should have been allowed to die were instead brought into hospital and sometimes ICU, and where they were subject to traumatic, unpleasant, and sometimes unnecessary interventions. With these "Western" experiences and being the first medical doctor in the extended family, perhaps I had inadvertently transformed into a self-centred soloist, a "holier than thou" crusader, or a colonialist with a mission.

Was I deaf to the relational aspects of death clearly demonstrated within the extended family? Or should I have asserted my way of making explicit 嫲嫲's wishes towards the end of life? Could I have trusted the healthcare providers to be realistic with 嫲嫲's care? Or was I right in insisting on a DNACPR to avoid assumptions? How do we navigate an increasingly medicalised, death-denying world and still uphold ancient wisdom around death and dying?

These questions don't have straightforward answers but expose the dissonance between the expectation of a "normal death" in traditional culture and the perceived desire to extend life so prevalent in healthcare. It challenges me as a physician to find some balance between what I experienced with 嫲嫲 and my professional expertise of keeping patients alive. It encourages me to seek personalised decisions for individual patients. It reminds me of the many immeasurable variables of life and death that extend far beyond the confines of healthcare. I am thankful that there was a beautiful cadence to 嫲嫲's life. It could have ended quite differently.

---

[65] Sallnow L, Smith R, Ahmedzai SH, Bhadelia A, Chamberlain C, Cong Y, et al. Report of the Lancet Commission on the Value of Death: bringing death back into life. The Lancet. 2022;399(10327):837-84.

Up to 90% of people in the UK want to die at home in the company of loved ones, but only 50% end up with that fate.[66] Most people instead end up dying in hospitals or nursing homes, and some in ICUs or hospices. The last year of life is also the most expensive. Up to 60% of lifetime health expenditure is spent in the last year of life, and not infrequently on investigations, therapies and treatments which are uncomfortable, poorly tolerated, and ultimately futile. While intensive care can make a difference for some people (as demonstrated by some of the stories in this book), for others, it is unlikely to lengthen meaningful survival. Many patients who have chronic, progressive conditions may become critically ill towards the end stages of their diseases. However, as many of these conditions progress, the likelihood of survival from critical illness diminishes.

Although many patients know that their health is deteriorating, few engage in conversations about their priorities and preferences before the onset of critical illness. Healthcare professionals are guilty of avoidance, too. When Maria, my friend who was suffering from a terminal disease, tried to speak to her specialist about putting an advanced care plan in place, she was told not to worry, and that the medications should help her. Maria wanted to discuss her priorities, knowing that her disease could cause her to lose mental capacity unpredictably at some stage. Instead, the specialist thought she was giving up altogether. Her ideas and concerns were not explored. An opportunity was missed to address fears. The door leading to preparation for death was closed. Unfortunately, Maria's family was also unwilling to engage with her in discussions about dying.

Conversations

Maria wanted to discuss an advanced care plan. The NHS describes Advanced Care Planning as "the voluntary process of person-centred discussion between an individual and their care providers about their preferences and priorities for their future care." It recognises the rapid development of advanced medical

---

[66] Curie M. A Place for Everyone - What stops people from choosing where they die? : Marie Curie; [Available from: https://www.mariecurie.org.uk/policy/a-place-for-everyone.

technologies capable of sustaining life, but at huge costs to individuals and the healthcare systems, without certainty of success.

Advanced care plans may include a resuscitation decision, but do not stop there. Good plans provide a brief overview of an individual's life, a succinct summary of their priorities, and what they might want should they lose the capacity to communicate, such as the *What Matters Most* charter, explored in the final pages of this book. These plans form narratives that can act as a roadmap for professionals when making complex decisions with uncertain risks and benefits. They give permission to move away from the pursuit of longevity at all costs and invite consideration of the relational aspects of life and death, just like Paul Kalanithi's supportive care, 嫲嫲's refusal of a pacemaker, and, in 2022, the death of Queen Elizabeth II.

Queen Elizabeth, knowing she was ageing and getting frailer, chose to move to Balmoral Palace during her last days to spend time with the family. She had planned it all beforehand with an advanced care plan (as do all members of the royal family). On the 8th of September 2022, when the Queen died comfortably at home, in the company of loved ones, many commented on how she had a "good" death. There are many reasons why people thought of it as "good". She was in control and realistic. She was comfortable, with her family, and in a familiar place.

Clearly, not everyone can be in control of their deaths. Sometimes, due to completely unforeseen circumstances (as with many stories in this book), intensive care is required before advanced care plans are made. At these points, death may not be certain, and there are usually reasonable chances of survival. Intensive care maximises those chances. Sadly, some never recover, and death becomes inevitable. These deaths are rarely "normal" and unlike what Mannix described in her book. Many interventions in intensive care, as detailed throughout this book, are a far cry from the preferred places and circumstances of death for most. However, it does not mean that such deaths are all undignified. In these situations, the initial time in intensive care may provide a "warning shot" for families, allowing time and space for exploration, reflection, and reconnection. Despite the circumstances, many families are thankful for this time, spending it holding hands with their loved one, having conversations with each other and reminiscing, oftentimes speaking to their loved ones even if they are sedated, semi-conscious, or comatose.[67] Therefore, even though the circumstances may not have been what the individual might have wanted, the relational aspects of death can still be reclaimed in the ICU.

During the Christmas after the Queen's death, my family and I listened to J.S. Bach's *Weihnachts Oratorium* as we usually do during advent. I was reminded of 嫲嫲's death, where the tension between traditional culture and medicine seemed to resolve as expected only because of favourable circumstances. I thought of Maria and the ongoing disconnects between the expectations of individuals and their healthcare providers. I considered Queen Elizabeth II and how she was an exemplar of what many people think of as a good way to die. Then, I reflected on the oratorio's fundamental narrative, which is exceptionally human – of the fragility of life, the certainty of death, and the hope of life after,

"Full of joy… there when life is over."

The beautiful music, profound lyrics, unwavering faith, and deep passion within the oratorio make it a timeless classic. It has been reimagined dozens of times by countless orchestras and choirs over the years. Similarly, Bach's other works continue to feature in many concerts all over the world. That Bach's music transcends death reflects his genius. That they have been reimagined, refashioned, and reinvented make them ideal analogies for the broad range of approaches and unique circumstances we find ourselves in when thinking about critical illness, dying, and death.

So, whatever your preferences, I hope that your thoughts and conversations about death and dying will create something

---

[67] There is evidence that patients can often hear and perceive their loved ones during periods of sedation or reduced consciousness, and towards the end of life. The following two papers describe some of our understanding: Blundon EG, Gallagher RE, Ward LM. Electrophysiological evidence of preserved hearing at the end of life. Sci Rep. 2020;10(1):10336. Hupcey JE, Zimmerman HE. The need to know: experiences of critically ill patients. American journal of critical care. 2000;9(3):192.

beautifully hopeful for you and your loved ones. Don't just talk about death. Sing. Sing by yourself and sing with your loved ones. Sing with your dearest or with strangers. Acknowledge the dissonances. Allow the countermelodies of disagreements to wander and wind. Respond to the swells of emotion with harmonic resolution. Keep your rhythm steady so that the polyrhythms may eventually converge. Hold the notes till they harmonise. Fear not. Let your heart move with the music, and sing about death until your very own oratorio is complete.

23. Curtain Call

There is still much we don't know about intensive care. In 2014, the James Lind Alliance, supported by the National Institute for Health and Care Research, published the results of their Priority Setting Partnership in Intensive Care Medicine. This research exercise involved clinicians, researchers – and most importantly, patients – in deciding the top ten priorities for research in intensive care medicine.

Two of their top priorities were:
1. Who benefits most from intensive care, and how best to identify them and escalate their care early?
2. How best can we support survivors of critical illness and their loved ones?

Throughout this book, you will have discovered the ongoing uncertainties of the first priority. You might also have glimpsed the longer-term consequences of survival from critical illness for patients and their families. Unfortunately, we have a poor understanding of the socio-cultural factors that help determine how well people cope and how best to support them. But that is another book for another day.

In the meantime, some readers may wish to discuss their care priorities and preferences after the stories in this book. Thus, this curtain call will provide some guidance towards this end. There are several publicly available resources to help navigate such discussions, including:

- The *Art of Dying* website (St Mary's University)
- *Deciding Right* (Northern Cancer Alliance)
- Death cafes run throughout the UK which provide safe forums
- The *What Matters Most* charter

They all advocate a similar process: to encourage people to talk more about death and dying. Most try to be as open-ended as possible, recognising the range of personal wishes, religious inclinations, and cultural nuances which shape society. However, some campaigns, such as *Dignity in Dying* and *My Death My Decision,* more explicitly advocate for assisted dying, which is a topic beyond the scope of this book. In this closing chapter, I will focus on the *What Matters Most* charter.[68]

In *What Matters Most*, there are four principles:

1. These conversations are voluntary and can occur at any point.
2. Promoting a culture of openness about living as well as possible, even with life-limiting conditions.
3. Conversations should be centred on individuals and their loved ones, and not on healthcare.
4. To enable living well until death.

Whilst being voluntary, they are becoming increasingly necessary in the Western world. The heavy emphasis on individual autonomy and the tendency for healthcare professionals to pursue life seem to reinforce each other. This means that if healthcare professionals do not know the priorities of the patient, they are likely to lean towards prolonging life, even if it means a potentially poorer quality of life, rather than a more realistic approach.

In more traditional cultures, where there is a narrower spectrum of social norms, death tends to be normalised even amongst healthcare professionals. This means that the expectation of a "normal" death is more commonly shared between the lay public and healthcare staff. Thus, it is more likely that healthcare professionals assume a more realistic stance regarding life support interventions. However, this may change with the increasing availability and affordability of healthcare in many middle-income countries experiencing rapid economic growth. In these settings, cultural changes are unlikely to keep pace with medical progress, resulting in a similar situation to that discussed in the previous chapter. Therefore, it seems prudent to plan ahead in such countries, too.

Practically speaking, several questions are useful for people to consider within two broad categories. The first category revolves around what matters most and provides peace to an individual, as well as how these might be the same or different should the

---

[68] EOLCPartners. What Matters Conversations: End of Life Care Partners Think Tank; 2020 [Available from: https://www.whatmattersconversations.org/2020-charter.

person be ill or dying. Seeking to make the most of life, it acknowledges that life can sometimes be unpredictable, people may live with chronic conditions, and that each person is an individual. For example, an increasing number of people live with health issues throughout middle age, such as mental health illnesses, physical impairments, metabolic diseases, or neuromuscular conditions. Thankfully, most are resilient and able to not only cope and survive with these conditions but also to thrive. However, one person may be content living and being dependent on another person for care (for example, if they have already lived with a progressive neuromuscular disease, as in the chapter *The Three Sisters*). Another may find this an outcome worse than death (see the chapter *Spice*). Similarly, having family around – talking in a bustling environment – may be comforting to one, but another may prefer silence and solitude.

Thus, the answers in this category help health and care practitioners better understand the key priorities of an individual. Knowing the "what matters most" preferences of our patients can help us to humanise what can be a painful, distressing, and traumatic experience in the ICU. It can also help people be more comfortable during the process of dying, despite the circumstances in ICU, and regain some of the autonomy frequently taken away during critical illness. Some units can facilitate some of these priorities. For example, the 3Wishes project helps facilitate the final three wishes for critically ill patients who are going to die and who are able to communicate their preferences.[69,70] Requests for a fine meal, a cuddle with a pet, or even hand sculptures made with clay have been facilitated. I've helped some longer-stay patients visit the hospital gardens to get some fresh air, and my colleagues have brought in horses and dogs as animal-assisted therapy on their ICUs. Some other units employ musicians to play for patients, much like discussed in *Gymnopedie*.

---

[69] Many critically ill patients are sedated and ventilated, making it impossible to communicate with them about such wishes.

[70] Vanstone M, Neville TH, Clarke FJ, Swinton M, Sadik M, Takaoka A, et al. Compassionate End-of-Life Care: Mixed-Methods Multisite Evaluation of the 3 Wishes Project. Ann Intern Med. 2020;172(1):1-11.

The second broad category goes into further detail about individual care preferences. These questions more explicitly explore where someone prefers to be cared for if unwell or dying, and at what point they might not wish to be admitted to a healthcare facility for a variety of treatments. Preferred place of death seems easy to answer but is based on an imagined future which may or may not come true. Much like birth plans, which intrinsically contain some unpredictability, death plans may be subject to changes outside of one's control. Part of this links to the second part regarding escalation of care. This can be quite difficult to explore if one has limited experience or understanding of the capabilities of medicine. Some people may have had long and detailed discussions with their doctors around realistic treatment goals, particularly if they have progressive and life-limiting conditions. But most don't, even if they have spent many hours contemplating such issues. Some may even have spoken with loved ones about it. Allowing and encouraging these discussions may help clinicians better understand individual priorities.

Sometimes, clinicians actively avoid the topic. Some think discussing death is a sign of "giving up", such as with Maria in the previous chapter. Others struggle with the idea of dying themselves and thus do not feel confident in discussing it. Some specialists, for many years practising in their own professional sphere, get too invested in their patients and cannot entertain the thought of deterioration. Here, multidisciplinary teams and collaborative working can help deliver the best quality care in difficult and deteriorating circumstances.

Occasionally, patients themselves are unwilling to discuss death and dying. This is usually due to the false perception that the person with the illness does not want to discuss it (as in Mannix's example and summarised in the chapter *Beyond Bach*). Some patients are scared by the potential pain and suffering they might endure, but this is usually not the truth of what lies ahead, and Mannix provides her lifetime of experience that suggests the contrary. Still, at other times, families hinder such discussions.

Fortunately, healthcare professionals can help to document such priorities even if families might be unwilling to discuss them.[71]

Further questions in this category seek to plan ahead. They focus on future care preferences in the face of life-limiting illness. These include making a will, limitations of care (including what might or might not be appropriate or acceptable), and appointing a power of attorney. The answers to these questions not only help with care in the community, they can also help hospital clinicians decide if intensive care is appropriate in the first place, or, for that matter, if an admission to hospital is required. Today, modern medicine can ensure patients' physical sufferings are minimised towards the end-of-life. Usually, these strategies are not only better for patients but also more sustainable for the environment and healthcare system. Compared to the financial and environmental costs of intensive care, good quality community-based care is far cheaper and more sustainable. Indeed, many interventions can be put into place at home.

When one of my uncles was dying at home in Singapore after years of being bed-bound due to advanced dementia, palliative care nurses were able to set up a syringe pump to administer painkillers and trained his wife to operate it. This ensured he remained in a comfortable environment and received care from familiar loved ones rather than being taken into hospital. Even non-invasive ventilation and supplemental oxygen can sometimes be facilitated at home, provided several criteria are fulfilled. Such care ensures the place of death can be optimised, relational aspects of dying are prioritised, and physical discomforts are minimised.

Intensive care, much like the rest of healthcare, performs most effectively when the phrase "prevention is better than cure" is put into practice. Most of these gains are centred within community-based initiatives and population health approaches.[72]

---

[71] Of course, it is better if these preferences are known beforehand rather than relying on healthcare organisations, where there are often changes of staff, different levels of experience, competing priorities, and sometimes a lack of familiarity with processes.

[72] Tan MZY. 1948 healthcare: still appropriate today? Journal of the Royal Society of Medicine. 2023;0(0):01410768231214336.

When the general population is healthier, there is less need for intensive care. When deterioration is identified early and action taken, some critically ill patients can avoid the need for intensive care altogether. When priorities are known and decisions are made beforehand, care can be focused on upholding individual values.

By exposing the realities of intensive care in this book and encouraging individuals to take control through *What Matters Most* conversations, everyone benefits. Individuals and their families are able to maintain their autonomy and dignity as much as possible for as long as possible. Clinicians can provide more personalised care whilst making the best use of the limited resources we have and ensuring they are available to those who may benefit from it most. Healthcare leaders can design systems that are potentially more sustainable. Researchers and policymakers can focus more on the health inequalities that continue to plague our world. And the world itself, well, maybe it will start to heal, too.

The stage is now yours.

The COVID-19 supplement

During the COVID-19 pandemic, I became acutely aware of the difficulties of communicating with patients' families, particularly when ICUs restricted visitors. Working during the initial stages of the pandemic also reminded me of the fragility of human life. I reflected on these aspects in several pieces.

The first was a short piece entitled *Telephone Lament for Coronavirus,* which was picked up by BBC Radio 4.

On the back of this, I was commissioned to write and present a Lent Talk for 2021: an annual series broadcast on BBC Radio 4 where "six well-known people in their fields reflect on the passion of Christ."

In between those two, I entered the piece *Critical but Stable* to the Doctors for the NHS essay competition under the theme "What lessons should we learn from the COVID-19 pandemic?"

These pieces form a significant part of my experiences during the COVID-19 pandemic. They also represent how the humanistic and relational aspects of health continue to be important, particularly during critical illness. They are thus reproduced here as a recognition of the pandemic's impact on intensive care medicine and a reminder that it still only forms part of the entire specialty and its history.

24. Telephone Lament for Coronavirus

In the style of Stevie Wonder's
"I just called to say I love you."

I just called, to say... your husband was admitted to the intensive care unit.

I sensed your shock even over the telephone. I realised you had only left for home a few hours earlier. I wondered if you imagined that he would be the unfortunate 10-15% of COVID-19 patients needing intensive care. I wondered if you knew that it took several consultants to decide to bring him to the intensive care unit. Perhaps you couldn't see the fear behind the flimsy masks of the emergency physicians: fear both for your husband, and for their own health.

I just called, to say... that he was stable on the breathing machine, with medications to keep him asleep.

I wondered if you realised "stable" still referred to needing near the maximal safe limit of pressure generated by the ventilator to drive air into the lungs. "Stable" meant he needed double or triple the fraction of oxygen available in normal air. "Stable" meant four different medications to keep him asleep to control his breathing, each with their own side effects.

Would you be less reassured by the term "stable" if you saw the multiple artificial lines inserted into your beloved husband, from the breathing tube to the plastic lines in his neck? From a small arterial catheter in his wrist to the larger urinary one in his bladder?

I just called, to ask... if you were alright yourself?

I wondered if you realised we healthcare workers also struggled to take care of ourselves. After all, many of our loved ones are of similar ages, with similar co-morbidities and health conditions as your husband. We couldn't help imagining our own loved ones in similar positions. We harboured the constant fear of bringing the virus back to our families. Like you, the lack of social gatherings impaired our resilience. We found solace in sources aplenty: prayer, meditation, books, exercise, gossip, dark humour, chocolate, alcohol… the list spiralled downwards. Our traditional knowledge and protocols were questioned, our prognostic methods challenged, our patience tested, and the gaping flaws in our systems revealed. Yet we looked outward and sought to care rather than to be cared for.

I just called, to say… it was too early to tell how he would fare in this disease process.

I wondered if you realised your husband would spend more than a couple of days on the ventilator, and that the mortality rates from ICUs around the country were hovering around 50% [during the initial stages of the pandemic]. Of all our prognostic methods and advanced technologies, his fate may as well be determined by a flip of a coin.

I wondered if you sensed the discomfort in my voice; the need to provide life-changing information over the phone. I wondered if you were shifting in your seat as much as I was, gripped by the realisation that the next fortnight would determine if your husband would live to see your face again. I felt disappointed for not being able to offer a tissue or a hand to hold over the phone when you broke into tears.

I just called, to say… his breathing was getting worse.

When I told you we had put him face-down to help his breathing, I wondered if you realised this took seven trained members of staff about an hour to perform safely. As I explained the ebb and flow of patient journeys in intensive care, I was thankful you could not see my head in my hands. Like many colleagues, I felt discouraged by the lack of improvement in other patients, just like your husband. I felt disheartened by the prolonged course of the disease, which tested our patience. I felt demoralised: the years of training and experience seemed meaningless in the face of a novel contagion.

I just called, to say… he had a sudden cardiac arrest.

I wondered no longer. I needed only to be sorry.

Sorry that the virus affected your husband's heart. Sorry that despite our best efforts, we were unable to resuscitate him successfully. Sorry that you could not be with him during his last hours. Sorry that you never met anyone from the team that took care of him. Sorry that while his death was consistent with the 5-10% overall mortality rate, he was still 100% of your life.

I just called, to say, how much we cared
I just called, to say, I'm sorry...
And we meant it from the bottom of our hearts.

[First broadcast on BBC Radio 4 on 25th April 2020.]

25. Critical but Stable

"Stable" from the Latin "stabilis",
from the base word "stare" meaning "to stand".

In the early stages of the COVID-19 pandemic, many ICUs severely restricted visitors. The reason was valid: minimise human contact and the transmission of infection could be controlled. As a result, many patient updates, which would normally have been carried out at the bedside or during a physical visit, needed to be done over the telephone. During this time, many of my colleagues (including myself) would use the word "stable" during our telephone updates with relatives.

Patients maintained on the same amount of life support were described as "stable", even if this involved high levels of oxygen, ventilators, or potent drugs. Indeed, most ICU patients with COVID-19 required heart or lung support and were, therefore, by definition, unstable. Why, then, did most of our telephone updates contain the word "stable"? Why did we struggle to describe the precarious situations our patients found themselves in? Why were we unable to balance the need to provide hope and convey severity to already distressed relatives?

Before COVID-19, I thought little about using the word "stable" in critically ill patient updates. After all, we are accustomed to the word. Phrases such as "your *[insert chronic disease]* is well under control" or "your *[biomarker or clinical measurement]* is stable with the medications" pervade medical lingo, particularly when chronic conditions are concerned. Think about patients who are diabetic and well-controlled for many years or those who experience no symptoms but take multiple medications for high blood pressure. We are used to hearing about stability and control. Stability is associated with longevity and health.

On a wider scale, society places an automatic value on the word "stable". Stable leadership was quoted as a key factor in successful responses to COVID-19 containment. Countries like Singapore and New Zealand, well-known for political stability, were recognised as positive role models during the pandemic, with low baseline levels and subdued spikes of infections.[73,74] But other stable governments in Europe, such as the UK and Germany, struggled to control the spread of the disease. In contrast, some fragile states in Africa and Asia-Pacific that were predicted to perform poorly actually fared better than expected.[75]

Psychologist Michele Gelfand argued for culture as a key characteristic of success since political stability was clearly not a determinant.[76] She asserted that "tight" cultures with law-abiding inhabitants managed to limit COVID-19's spread, while "looser" cultures struggled to contain the virus despite restrictive infection control measures and more resources. It was perhaps one of many factors that contributed to pandemic performance.

With such weight placed on a single word, and the control it portrays, it is little wonder intensivists are known to use phrases such as "critical but stable". Yet, such ambiguous terms and vague phrases have been the source of interdisciplinary misunderstandings, as noticed even before COVID-19.[77] World-renowned intensivist and researcher Jean-Louis Vincent reflected on an anecdote in 2019 where one colleague described a patient's condition as "stable", which in turn provided a sense of hope for the patient's loved ones. The term carried a positive connotation for the family, even though the patient was still incredibly ill and required multiple drugs to support his heart. In this case, "stable" described a lack of clinical deterioration. But the longer someone spends on ICU (even without clinical deterioration), the lower their chances of recovery. So, "stable" actually gave the family false hope.

---

[73] Farrer M. New Zealand's COVID-19 response the best in the world, say global business leaders. The Guardian. 2020.

[74] Lewis R, Yap J. COVID-19: The response in Singapore: Nuffield Trust; 2020 [Available from: https://www.nuffieldtrust.org.uk/news-item/covid-19-the-response-in-singapore.

[75] Andrews M, Eissa N, Bousso A. COVID-19 and the State Fragility Trap London: London School of Economics and Political Science; 2020 [Available from: https://www.lse.ac.uk/iga/Maryam-Forum/Maryam-Forum-Launch-sessions/COVID-19-and-the-State-Fragility-Trap.

[76] Gelfand M. Rule Makers, Rule Breakers: How Tight and Loose Cultures Wire Our World: Scribner; 2018.

[77] Vincent JL, Cecconi M, Saugel B. Is this patient really "(un)stable"? How to describe cardiovascular dynamics in critically ill patients. Crit Care. 2019;23(1):272.

When used in patient conversations like this, the term "stable" simply fails to address the long and arduous journeys of critically ill patients or the various levels of support they need to survive. Moreover, over the telephone, families lose the usual visual and environmental input with which to frame such conversations. Without seeing the lines and tubes, hearing the multiple alarms, or feeling the cold, clammy skin of near-death, families struggle to appreciate the severity of the clinical situation (see also the chapter *Painting an ICU*). In other words, as reflected in communication studies, non-verbal cues convey far more information than speech can.[78]

The fact is stability is not a key feature of critical illness trajectories. Most patients' admissions to critical care are characterised by instability, either from cardiovascular, respiratory, or metabolic systems.[79] Instability does not simply disappear upon discharge either. Many ICU survivors face long-term complications, lingering labels, and societal stigma.[80] These include mental health issues, physical disabilities, cognitive impairments, and other problems.

Trajectories towards the end of life may provide further evidence to refute the stability narrative we project. These are understood in at least three distinct functional trajectories: sudden decline, intermittent episodic deterioration, and prolonged dwindling.[81] With sudden decline, patients are relatively well until severe illness causes a short spell of deterioration prior to death. The intermittent episodic trajectory describes a slow decline in physical condition, punctuated with occasional severe episodes of illness from which the patient makes a good recovery. The prolonged dwindling trajectory

---

[78] Piazza O, Cersosimo G. Communication as a basic skill in critical care. J Anaesthesiol Clin Pharmacol. 2015;31(3):382-3.

[79] ICNARC. ICNARC report on COVID-19 in critical care: England, Wales and Northern Ireland 10 May 2021 London: Intensive Care National Audit and Research Centre; 2021 [Available from: https://www.icnarc.org/Our-Audit/Audits/Cmp/Reports.

[80] Missel M, Bernild C, Westh Christensen S, Dagyaran I, Kikkenborg Berg S. The marked body - a qualitative study on survivors embodied experiences of a COVID-19 illness trajectory. Scand J Caring Sci. 2021.

[81] Murray SA, Kendall M, Boyd K, Sheikh A. Illness trajectories and palliative care. BMJ. 2005;330(7498):1007-11.

describes a slow, progressive decline in physical condition over a prolonged period towards the end of life. While all three trajectories may feature periods of seemingly relative calm, there is still an overall decline and growing fragility, which eventually leads to death. Even with the intermittent episodic deteriorating trajectory, there continues to be an impression of sudden deterioration towards the end of life.

Anushua Gupta is a GP, mother, and survivor of COVID-19. When she was critically ill, she was put on Extra-Corporeal Membrane Oxygenation (ECMO).[82] She teetered on the brink of death for many weeks, but the word "stable" was frequently used during update conversations. Unable to visit, her husband struggled to imagine her progress (or lack thereof). He was told about her physiological variables and biomarkers over the phone, but these can only convey a limited amount of information about a patient's condition, particularly in ICU, where active manipulation of organ systems can provide a false sense of security. If Anushua's husband, himself a GP, felt unable to comprehend the severity of critical illness based on the terminology used, then what hope did the non-medical public have?

Beyond mere communication, the absence of family during a critical care stay further destabilises the entire healthcare journey. Family absence probably exacerbates the already problematic "post-intensive care syndrome" suffered by ICU survivors and their families.[83] In contrast, the presence of family has been shown to be a contributor to both physiological and psychological well-being and recovery.[84] Such human connection is all the more important with the depersonalisation associated with Personal Protective Equipment (PPE) used in ICU during

---

[82] Gupta A. COVID-19 and extracorporeal membrane oxygenation: experiences as a patient, general practitioner, wife and mother. Anaesth Rep. 2021;9(1):101-5.

[83] Newcombe V, Baker T, Burnstein R, Tasker R, Menon D. Clinical communication with families in the age of COVID-19: a challenge for critical care teams BMJ Opinion: British Medical Journal; 2020 [Available from: https://blogs.bmj.com/bmj/2020/08/11/clinical-communication-with-families-in-the-age-of-covid-19-a-challenge-for-critical-care-teams/.

[84] Page P. Critical illness trajectory for patients, families and nurses - a literature review. Nurs Crit Care. 2016;21(4):195-205.

the COVID-19 pandemic. The anonymity, ambiguity and androgyny associated with full PPE further limited the humanisation of provider-patient relationships,[85] reversing the many years it has taken to move away from a rigidly paternalistic system.

So, if "stable" is insufficient to describe ICU patients, how can intensivists better navigate such conversations? Several months into the pandemic, many ICUs adopted video-based telecommunication technologies like FaceTime and Zoom. They helped mitigate the lack of visual and environmental input during family communications. Families who could see the clinical state of their loved ones could better comprehend the severity of illness. Such technologies also allowed healthcare professionals to convey both verbal and non-verbal information. But even these were compromises.

Current international family-centred guidelines recommend "formal, structured communication to ensure that clinical decision making is informed by a shared understanding of diagnosis and prognosis and patient goals and preferences".[86] Clearly, face-to-face encounters can meet such recommendations far better than any video call. The use of frameworks can also help clinicians maximise the effectiveness of family communications. An example is the Serious Illness Conversation (SIC) guide.[87] Like other guides, they follow a generic format, which begins with building rapport, establishing the purpose of the conversation, and probing for information. After this comes the difficult part of sharing the prognosis. Because this is often difficult to predict accurately, the SIC guide advises the use of "wish...sorry" or "hope...worry" statements. This provides an honest exploration of the fine balances we are often required to

---

[85] Brown-Johnson C, Vilendrer S, Heffernan MB, Winter S, Khong T, Reidy J, et al. PPE Portraits-a Way to Humanize Personal Protective Equipment. J Gen Intern Med. 2020;35(7):2240-2.

[86] Davidson JE, Aslakson RA, Long AC, Puntillo KA, Kross EK, Hart J, et al. Guidelines for Family-Centered Care in the Neonatal, Pediatric, and Adult ICU. Crit Care Med. 2017;45(1):103-28.

[87] Pasricha V, Gorman D, Laothamatas K, Bhardwaj A, Ganta N, Mikkelsen ME. Use of the Serious Illness Conversation Guide to Improve Communication with Surrogates of Critically Ill Patients. A Pilot Study. ATS Sch. 2020;1(2):119-33.

strike. Following this, a further exploration of individual priorities, fears, and sources of support enable a holistic approach to wellbeing, including spirituality. Finally, a summary, recommendation, and check for understanding can draw the conversation to a close, even if there are sometimes no concrete answers to questions. Such structured communication increases the understanding and sense of control for families and provides greater satisfaction for the clinician.

In addition, the use of imagery may be helpful for visualisation. For example, a stringed instrument requires tension for appropriate sound production. Too tight and a string will snap, but too loose and it fails to produce a sound. So, too, can our interventions be framed, particularly in ICU, where we constantly tread fine lines between risk and benefit. Other dynamic processes such as sine waves, roller coasters, vortices and spirals have all been described in ICU patient literature.[88,89] By performing such facilitative or collaborative communication, we can further strive to empower family participation in critical care, improving overall physician and patient satisfaction, and raising the overall standard of care.[90]

In the end, perhaps the most striking rebuttal of the stability narrative in intensive care comes from the etymology of the word "stable". The fact that intensive care units were filled with prone or supine patients suffering from multi-systemic diseases, and reliant on machines to maintain basic physiology, clearly indicated their inability "to stand". The numerous waves and multiple variants which overwhelmed global healthcare systems during the pandemic brought the medical profession to its knees.

---

[88] Sturmey G, Wiltshire M. Patient perspective: Gordon Sturmey and Matt Wiltshire. BMJ. 2020;369:m1814.

[89] Kirchhoff KT, Walker L, Hutton A, Spuhler V, Cole BV, Clemmer T. The vortex: families' experiences with death in the intensive care unit. Am J Crit Care. 2002;11(3):200-9.

[90] Arnold R, Judith Nelson, Thomas Prendergast, Lillian Emlet, Elizabeth Weinstein, Amber Barnato, et al. Educational Modules for the Critical Care Communication (C3) Course - A Communication Skills Training Program for Intensive Care Fellows Los Angeles: UCLA Health; 2010 [Available from: https://www.uclahealth.org/palliative-care/Workfiles/Educational-Modules-Critical-Care-Communication.pdf.

The countless lives lost ran the human spirit into the ground. The COVID-19 pandemic was anything but stable.

So, I ditched the "stable" during COVID-19 and embraced the fragility that it exposed, for it is through fragility that we continue to hope. Through humility, we practise the selflessness needed to care for the critically ill. It is through instability that the human spirit clambers, climbs, and conquers, just like a patient's recovery trajectory, until humanity stands undefeated.

"Where there is love for man,
there is also love for the art of medicine" - Hippocrates

[3rd prize winner of the Doctors for the NHS essay competition in 2021. First published in Intensive Care Medicine journal in March 2022: Tan MZY. Critical but stable—critical care communication in the COVID-19 pandemic**. Intensive Care Medicine (Springer Nature). 2022;48:1127–9. Available from: [https://link.springer.com/article/10.1007/s00134-022-06675-4] Used with permission.]

26. A Letter to Lydia

Dear Lydia,

Sleeping peacefully in my arms, you are our ray of sunshine, our bundle of joy, our beacon of hope. Outside our embrace, however, the world seems far less hopeful. See, you were born in the middle of a pandemic – COVID-19 – which has ravaged our social landscape, torn apart the fabric of our society, and robbed us of many things we have taken for granted.

Papa is an anaesthetics and intensive care doctor. He has been caring for the sickest patients, whose bodies are unable to support their own lives. Your silent breaths are a tranquil breeze compared to theirs. They all need help from a machine for what you do so effortlessly. Your scent, and that milky breath, they are an intoxicating escape from the fetid stench of near-death worn by the critically ill. As I hold your fragile frame in my arms, the warmth re-ignites a flame within me, daily extinguished by the tepid, diaphoretic skin I touch through gloved hands. Some may remain in this state for weeks, organ by organ slowly succumbing to the death grip of infection, all while we try to support the basic functions of life. You see, almost half of the patients I see will die of this dreadful disease.

When you were in the womb, Mama and I argued about whether I should stay apart from the family. Several colleagues had already made that decision. Some stayed apart; others sent the kids to their grandparents. We were all afraid of bringing the virus home from work. But I could not face it. I did not know how to cope if I could not come home to Mama and your sister Miriam. I needed to hug, to touch, and to cry with them. So, I made sure I took extra sets of clothes to work. I showered with an antiseptic solution after each shift. I even changed my socks and underwear before I cycled home. I went straight to the bathroom to wash my hands when I got home. Only then did I kiss Mama and Miriam. It was strange, but a minor sacrifice compared to many families who stayed apart.

A few weeks before you were born, I stood outside a bay and looked at two particular patients. Both were ventilated by machines. Both needed multiple drugs. Both were fighting for

their lives. One was a junior doctor. His name was Paul. He was
a few years younger than me. He was working on a respiratory
ward looking after COVID-19 patients. He did not have full
protective equipment, so became a victim himself. The other
patient was John. He was my age. He was a father of two, just
like me. Taking care of a critically ill patient the same age as me
is disconcerting. Taking care of a colleague on ICU is
excruciating. Daily, I was reminded of my own fragile existence.
I was confronted by the sheer injustice of this disease, its
seeming irreverence for age, class or health status, its uninhibited
pattern of transmission and its propensity to cause such
disruption.

Many colleagues are already burnt out from the stress, the
uncertainties, and the unrelenting torrent of critically ill patients.
I, too, have suffered. Mama will tell you how I was grumpy for
days. I lost my temper and shouted at your sister. My jaw began
to hurt and lock from stress. I struggled to eat. Many things
seemed meaningless, and I found little joy, even at home.
Indeed, the uncertainties are numerous. Questions relate to
admission, like: Who should come to ICU? What are their
chances of survival? What might their quality of life be after
survival? Other questions are based around treatment. Should we
support this organ? What is the balance between risk and benefit
for an invasive procedure? How can we prevent complications
from our artificial manipulation of physiology? Still other
questions relate to communication. Should we allow visitors?
How do we convey severity without instilling panic? How can we
provide hope without false optimism?

In the Christmas video from the Intensive Care Society last
year, ICU survivors shared their messages of thanks for the ICU
teams who saved their lives. It was a powerful reminder of why
we continue to do what we do. Through their encouragement,
these survivors gave us hope, urging us to keep going, giving us a
glimpse of life beyond near-death, and providing us with
sustenance through what many of us perceive as our professional
wilderness.

I realised that hope was there in the midst of the uncertainties.
It was not just the sophisticated machinery or the complex
monitoring. Hope was standing beside each of the patients' beds.

Hope was the nurse, the healthcare assistant, and the doctor. It was the sore upon our noses, the band across our foreheads and the sweat on our scrubs, all from the protective equipment we donned. Hope was possessing the perseverance to care despite the scars in our heads, the bitter taste of injustice, and the nails in our hearts. And it was why we went home after each shift to a full or empty house.

You will be at least a year old before you even get to see your grandparents. I know they are yearning to hold you, but they are overseas. 爷爷 (yeye, grandpa) and 奶奶 (nainai, grandma) are in Singapore, and Opa and Oma are in Germany. The virus has caused severe travel restrictions, so they are unable to come. My patients' loved ones also long to see them again. The wife for her husband, the child for their parent, the parent for their child. They ache with longing. They wait, as Anatole Broyard suggested during his encounter with critical illness, "more intensely than a lover". Patiently, they hope once again to have and to hold. So, we wait as they wait, and we hope as they hope. For without faith and without hope, we would not accept our patients.

It is because of hope that we contravene the Hippocratic oath to "do no harm". We insert the needles into wrists for precise blood pressure monitoring, and larger drains into chests to release pressure on the lungs. We force long tubes into throats and make holes into necks for tracheostomies. We use potent drugs which sometimes cause terrifying alterations of consciousness. Our methods may seem brutal, but it is sometimes through such life-sustaining treatment that recovery is facilitated.

For most loved ones, their wait is not indefinite, but the reunion is often framed within unexpected contexts. As TS Eliot puts it, "Their beginning was their end, and their end was their beginning".

Paul recovered from COVID-19 and was eventually discharged from ICU and then from the hospital. He went home to be with his parents. But the end of his illness was the beginning of another journey. For the scars of survivorship are not always visible. ICU survivors take months, if not years, to regain physical function, rebuild relationships, reorganise priorities and recover from psychological trauma. John's reunion

245

with his wife was due to a more divergent reason. He was dying. While we stopped visitors to ICU due to the risk of spreading infection, we also recognised the unmeasurable agony of dying alone. So, they reunited; till death did them part. The beginning of his illness journey was his end. And as he breathed his last, his end was also a beginning.

Left behind was the widowed mother of two, who had her own grief to overcome and a new chapter of life to navigate. As a secondary victim of critical illness, her challenges were not dissimilar to those of other ICU survivors. She had to rebuild her own life. Her relationships would never be the same. She had to continue to love her children when the love of her life was extinguished.

I do not know why John died and Paul did not. We still do not fully understand the susceptibility to symptoms nor the predisposition to severity. But even though I am confronted by death every day, I am also surrounded by hope. Hope that is not confined to the beginning or the end of an illness. As I reflect on the sacrifices made by healthcare workers, and those made by patients, I am reminded of the long history of personal sacrifice within medicine. The Byzantine Christians, disregarding their own safety, cared for victims of the plague. This, along with the formation of hospices, developed into the specialty of palliative care. Henry Dunant, who witnessed the horrors of the battle of Solferino, spent his wealth and energy during later life campaigning for humanitarianism, culminating in the formation of the Red Cross. Within this pandemic, the hundreds of healthcare workers who have died from COVID-19 stand testament to the undying hope we hold for a better future.

Healthcare professionals continue to work despite the adversities, uncertainties and insufficiencies. Scientists have had years' worth of work and funding disrupted, but their efforts – despite this forced directional change – have brought us hope in the vaccine. Numerous drug trials have already identified several treatment options to reduce mortality. Though the deaths of patients are etched in my memory, I carry on, knowing that our work is one of hope. Each patient I admit, I hope, along with their loved ones, that they will live. But for those who do not, I echo what the late Professor Jay Katz wrote, "We cannot resurrect the dead, but we can learn from their suffering".

My dear Lydia, the world you were born into may seem daunting. It is often confusing, occasionally frustrating and sometimes seems hopeless. You will sometimes feel pain, and you might endure suffering, but life really isn't "the curtain descends, everything ends, too soon, too soon". On finishing a shift one morning as the on-call anaesthetist for maternity, I became acutely aware of the hope which shines through birth. Through your birth, we left behind the sufferings and sacrifices of pregnancy. We moved on from the fact that Papa was not allowed to attend antenatal appointments or scans. We rejoice in the gift of new life. In the global narrative of many endings, you are indeed a new beginning. And as Easter approaches, remember that the darkest ending was also followed by the brightest beginning. So, as you grow up, never forget the sacrifices made so that we may live and have a better future. Never forget the blood of Christ that gives us hope. Never forget the light which shines through the darkness and is not overcome by it.

Love, Papa.

[First broadcast for BBC Radio 4 Lent Talks on 24th February 2021 and shortlisted for the Sandford St Martin Broadcasting Awards 2022.]

Other Books from the Publisher

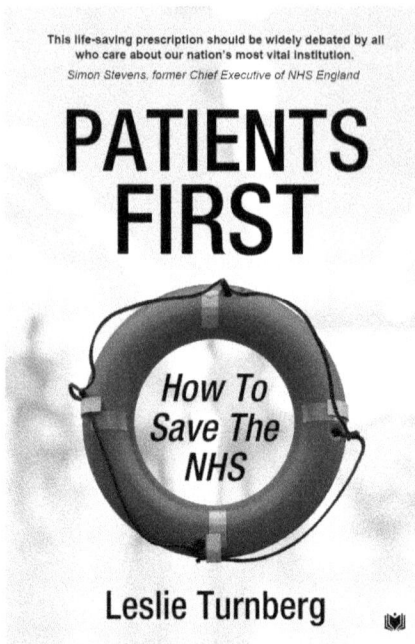

Patients First

This life-saving prescription should be widely debated by all who care about our nation's most vital institution.
Simon Stevens, former Chief Executive of NHS England

PATIENTS FIRST

How To Save The NHS

Leslie Turnberg

In *Patients First*, Leslie Turnberg, former President of the Royal College of Physicians, focuses on the needs of NHS patients and the staff who care for them. Shining a light on the many challenges facing the NHS and Primary and Social Care, and resisting any suggestion of yet another wholesale reorganisation, he pinpoints where and how to improve outcomes.

It is clear that the caring services must change and a patient-centred model – where a disillusioned workforce is brought back into satisfying and contented employment – should be the aim. Chapters on Social care and Primary Care come first, as so much in secondary care is dependent on them. Chapters on Public Health, Mental Health, and Maternity Care provide examples of where significant improvements may be gained. Further chapters on Trust in the NHS, Research, and Funding follow.

Patients First is a must-read for anyone interested in an NHS action plan for the future.

Lord Turnberg carefully takes the temperature of an ailing NHS. His life-saving prescription should be widely debated by all who care about our nation's most vital institution. **Lord Simon Stevens, former Chief Executive of NHS England**

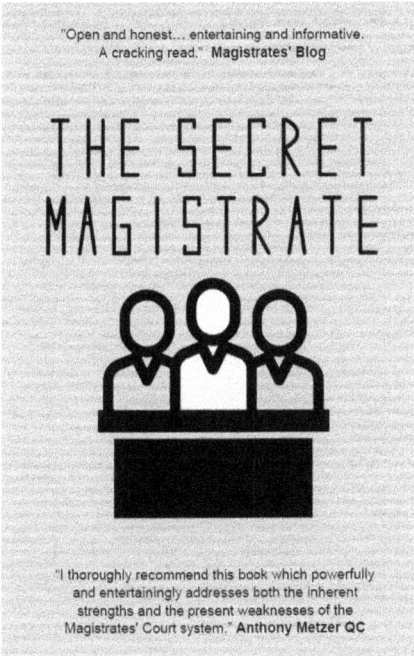

The Secret Magistrate

THE SECRET MAGISTRATE

Every criminal case starts in a magistrates' court, and most end there. Last year, the 14,000 magistrates of England & Wales dealt with almost 1.4 million cases.

But, what exactly does a magistrate do, who are they, and how are they recruited and trained? Are they out-of-touch and unrepresentative, or still fit for purpose with a role to play in today's increasingly sophisticated and complex judicial system?

The Secret Magistrate takes the reader on an eye-opening, behind-the-scenes tour of a year in the life of an inner-city magistrate. Chapters cover a variety of cases including the disqualified driver who drove away from court, the Sunbed Pervert, and Fifi the Attack Chihuahua.

Master Your Chronic Pain: A Practical Guide

Chronic pain is a huge problem. It is estimated that between one third and one half of the adult population in the UK live with pain. In turn, many people struggle to manage their pain; they report that it affects nearly every aspect of their lives, and that they feel held captive by it.

A Practical Guide

MASTER YOUR CHRONIC PAIN

Dr Nicola Sherlock

Furthermore, the emotional impact of pain has been increasingly recognised, and it is recommended that treatments for chronic pain no longer rely on medication alone. However, it is difficult to find relatable, easy-to-understand information on the non-medical aspects of pain management.

Master Your Chronic Pain adopts a holistic view of pain. Each chapter looks at a different aspect of pain management, from the benefits of mindfulness meditation to overcoming a fear of exercise to strategies for improving sleep. The emotional impact of pain is discussed, and practical tips for managing stress, worry, and low mood are given. Strategies for managing thoughts and emotions are explored, and the impact of pain on relationships is examined. This book uses principles from Acceptance and Commitment Therapy (ACT) which has been established as a highly effective therapeutic approach in the management of chronic pain.

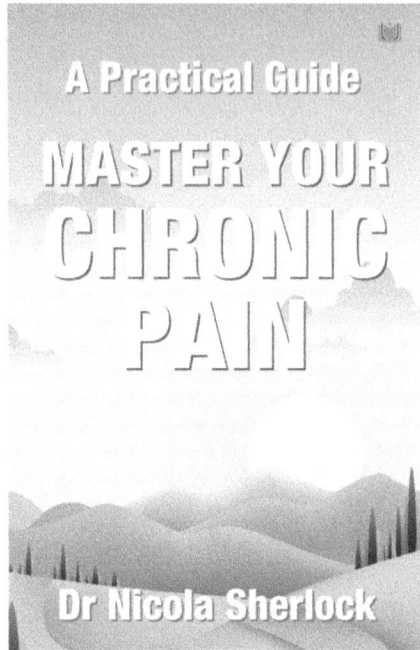

www.ingramcontent.com/pod-product-compliance
Lightning Source LLC
Chambersburg PA
CBHW041733200326
41518CB00020B/2583